Abdominal Radiology

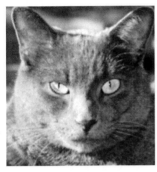

for the
Small Animal Practitioner

by
Judith A. Hudson, DVM, PhD, DipACVR
William R. Brawner, DVM, PhD, DipACVR
Merrilee Holland, DVM, MS, DipACVR
Margaret A. Blaik, DVM, MSc, DipACVR

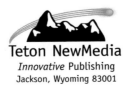

Teton NewMedia
Innovative Publishing
Jackson, Wyoming 83001

Executive Editor: Carroll C. Cann
Development Editor: Susan L. Hunsberger
Editor: Cynthia J. Roantree
Design & Layout: Anita B. Sykes

Teton NewMedia
P.O. Box 4833
Jackson, WY 83001
1-888-770-3165
www.tetonnm.com

PRINTED IN THE UNITED STATES OF AMERICA

ISBN # 1-893441-32-6

Print number 5 4 3 2

Library of Congress Cataloging-in-Publication Data

Abdominal radiology for the small animal practitioner / Judith A. Hudson... [et al.}
    p. ; cm.
  Includes bibliographical references.
  ISBN 1-893441-32-6 (alk. paper)
  1. Veterinary radiography. 2. Abdomen--Diseases--Diagnosis. I. Hudson, Judith A.,
1949-
  [DNLM: 1. Radiography, Abdominal--veterinary. 2. Animal Diseases--radiography. 3.
Radiography, Abdominal--methods. SF 757.8 A135 2001]
SF757.8 .A23 2001
636.7'089607572--dc21

                                                                      2001027971

Dedication

To my family (Bill, Mike, Patricia, Colleen, Joey) who surrounded me with love and tolerated long sessions with the computer.

To my father who inspired me.

To my friends and colleagues who supported me.

And...in memory of Wally. We miss you.

— Judy Hudson

To my wife, Jenny.

To my sons, Blue, Bo, and Michael.

— Bill Brawner

To my nephews, Gavin and Dalton.

And in memory of my sister, Joy.

— Merrilee Holland

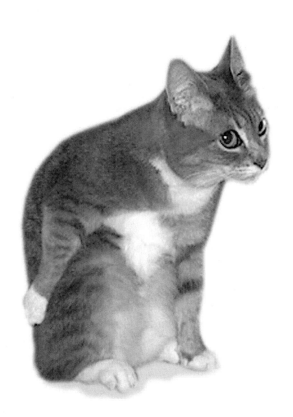

Preface

Interpretation of abdominal radiographs is complicated by the lack of contrast compared to other body systems. In the thorax, fluid-opaque structures such as the heart are clearly contrasted against the air-filled lungs. There is an obvious difference between the fluid-opaque muscles and the mineral-opaque bones of the musculoskeletal system. In the abdomen, however, virtually all structures are fluid-opaque and are recognizable only by the fat that surrounds them and by their relationship to surrounding organs. To be successful in interpretation, one needs to think in terms of opacities and must reconstruct a 3-dimensional picture from a 2-dimensional image.

It is the hope of this book to help the reader learn to transform a radiograph from a flat black and white picture to a 3-dimensional image with multiple shades of grey to visualization of the abdomen which it represents. This text will describe the normal appearance of the abdomen, ways in which the radiographic appearance changes to reflect disease, basic radiographic techniques, and common abdominal disorders. The text is meant to be a handy "cookbook" which can be quickly grabbed from the shelf rather than a comprehensive volume which would require intensive study. Many comprehensive texts have been used to compile this *Made Easy* book and they are gratefully listed in the Recommended Readings.

Judy Hudson

William Brawner

Merrilee Holland

Margaret Blaik

Table Of Contents

Section 1 Introduction and Radiographic Technique

Section 2 Normal Radiographic Anatomy of the Abdomen

Section 3 Peritoneal Cavity

Section 4 Intra-abdominal Masses

Section 5 Alimentary Tract

Section 6 Urinary Tract

Section 7 Reproductive Tract

Section 8 Anomalies

Recommended Readings

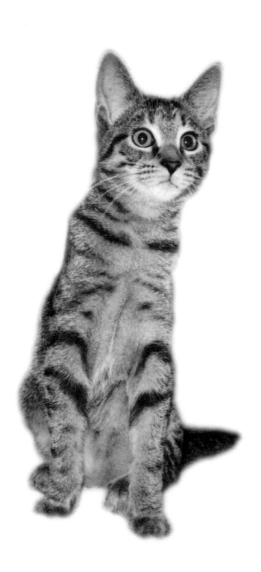

Section 1

Introduction and Radiographic Technique

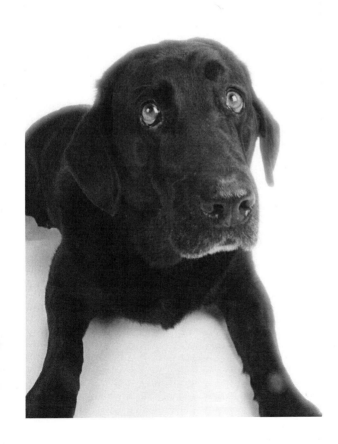

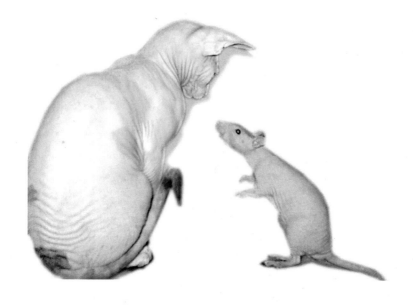

Introduction

The goals of this book are to help the reader acquire good techniques for making and interpreting radiographs of the abdomen, and to give the reader a good basic knowledge of special procedures available to gain additional diagnostic information. Although ultrasonography has added immeasurable diagnostic capability, abdominal radiography frequently can yield additional information by providing a panoramic view of the abdomen and by allowing examination of tissues hidden from the ultrasound beam by bone or gas.

Some Helpful Hints

The following icons are used in this book to indicate important concepts:

✓   Routine. This feature is routine, something you should know.

♥   Important. This concept strikes at the heart of the matter.

☙ Key. This concept is a key one and is necessary for full understanding.

💣 Stop. This statement appears to be simple but is more important than you might think.

⊙ A companion CD is available for purchase by calling 877-306-9793. The CD contains the full text, figures, and tables of this book formatted for easy search and retrieval. The CD symbol indicates that additional images of a topic are available on the CD.

Indications for Abdominal Radiography

✓ Vomiting
✓ Abdominal pain
✓ Regurgitation
✓ Palpable abdominal mass
✓ Diarrhea
✓ Hematuria/dysuria
✓ Tenesmus
✓ Herniations
✓ Rectal bleeding
✓ Suspected foreign body
✓ Staging of neoplasia
✓ Geriatric examination
✓ Others by clinical judgement

Role of Radiology in Patient Management

1. Diagnosis
   ✓ One of many diagnostic aids
   ✓ Expand or reduce differential diagnosis
   ✓ Precise diagnosis not always possible
2. Prognosis
3. Evaluate course of disease with or without therapy

Steps to Good Film Reading

1. Evaluate technical factors
2. Read the whole film
   ✓ Fight clinical bias
   ☙ Perform a systematic interpretation.

3. Describe the film in terms of roentgen or radiographic signs e.g., opacity, size, shape, position, margination, intraluminal, extraluminal

4. Assess signs and list differential diagnoses

5. What happens next?

Step 1: Technical Factors for Abdominal Radiography

✓ Proper preparation—fasting and enema if possible

✓ Adequate restraint

♥ Always two views (ventrodorsal or dorsoventral and lateral)

✓ Include diaphragm and pelvic inlet

✓ Use grid when abdomen is greater than 9 cm thick

Determine technique chart and be consistent.

✓ Make the exposure at the expiratory pause to avoid motion artifact.

Step 2: Using a System for Interpretation

Whether you use a regional or organ system approach is unimportant, but you must cover the entire film.

✓ In the regional approach, you read from the center out, from periphery in, or from side-to-side, or some other variation to cover all regions of the film.

✓ In the organ system approach, organs are listed and identified and unusual opacities are noted.

  ✓ Spine, caudal thorax, and other intra-abdominal structures should be examined first.

  ✓ It may be helpful to begin examination of the abdomen with large solid organs like the liver, spleen, kidneys, etc.

  ✓ Then identify visible portions of the GI tract.

  ✓ Mentally check off organs that are not usually seen and look for them.

  ✓ Look for unusual opacities that cannot be readily identified.

Abdominal Structures Normally Visualized on Survey Films

Stomach	Cecum
Urinary bladder	Sublumbar musculature
Duodenum	Spleen
Prostate gland	Vertebrae
Small intestines	Liver
Diaphragm	Caudal ribs
Colon	Kidneys
Body wall	Pelvis

Abdominal Structures Not Normally Visualized on Survey Films

Adrenal glands	Ovaries
Mesentery	Uterus
Mesenteric lymph nodes	Ureters
Omentum	Abdominal aorta
Pancreas	Abdominal vena cava
Gall bladder	

Step 3: Roentgen or Radiographic Signs

Signs should be recorded as a description of what you see, particularly things that are abnormal. Describe your findings in terms of opacity, size, shape, position, margins, and intraluminal/extraluminal.

✔ Do the organs have their expected relative opacity?

✔ Are any organs smaller or larger than usual?

✔ Do the organs have a normal shape?

✔ Are the organs in their normal position? A change in position could be caused by an adjacent organ being smaller or larger than usual or by displacement of the organ by congenital defects or trauma.

✔ Abnormal margins of an organ can indicate disease.

✔ In the abdomen, it may be important to note whether something is intraluminal or extraluminal.

Radiographic Opacity

☞ There are four distinct radiographic opacities of biologic materials:

GAS   FAT   FLUID   BONE

in order from least to most radiopaque.

♥ Remember that **METAL**, the fifth radiopaque opacity, is more radiopaque than all of these.

A Word About Radiographic Opacity

✓ Determined by chemical composition

✓ Absorption of x-rays is a factor of subject density and thickness

✓ X-rays will turn the film black

✓ Structures that absorb x-rays will be white or light grey – **radiopaque**

✓ Structures that do not absorb x-rays will be black or dark grey – **radiolucent**

☀ When two structures of the same opacity are in contact, the confluent borders cannot be distinguished (silhouette sign).

☀ If two structures are superimposed, their opacities will be added together creating a summation effect.

Abdominal Opacities

✓ The thorax has good subject contrast.

♥ All abdominal organs are fluid opaque, so subject contrast is poor.

☞ Fat surrounding organs allows serosal surfaces to be seen (Figure 1-1).

☀ If there is no fat (emaciation) or the animal is immature, serosal surfaces will not be seen, and the abdomen will appear as fluid-opaque (Figure 1-2).

☞ Intraluminal gas allows mucosal surfaces to be seen and permits identification of intestinal loops.

✓ Abnormal opacities help diagnose disease (e.g., foreign bodies, calculi).

✓ Subject contrast is best in fat or obese animals.

☀ The exception is when the animal is so large that excessive scatter causes a loss of detail.

Step 4: Differential Diagnoses

💣* There is seldom a single diagnosis.

✓ Make a list of differential diagnoses.

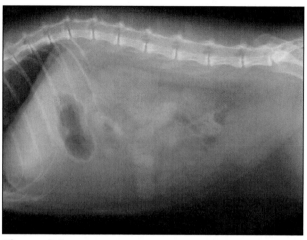

Figure 1-1
Lateral view of a fat cat that shows excellent serosal detail.

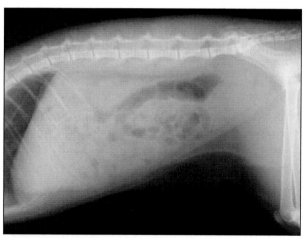

Figure 1-2
Lateral view of the cat in Figure 1-1 after a fractured jaw caused marked weight loss.

✓ Prioritize the list from the most to least likely diagnosis.

Step 5: What's Next?

✓ Additional views or contrast radiography

✓ Additional imaging procedures such as ultrasound, CT, MRI, or nuclear scintigraphy

✓ Additional diagnostic procedures other than imaging, such as cystocentesis, biopsy, or laparotomy.

✓ Are we ready to treat?

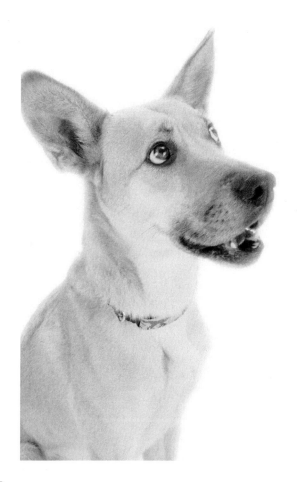

Section 2

Normal Radiographic Anatomy of the Abdomen

Viewing the Film

☛ Left and right lateral recumbent views are exposed with the patient in left or right lateral recumbency.

✓ By convention, lateral recumbent views are placed on the view box with the cranial aspect to the left.

✓ To correlate the left lateral recumbent view to gross anatomy (Figure 2-1):

> Mentally picture the animal on its left side with the head to the right of your mental image.

> Mentally remove the right chest wall.

> Using mental gymnastics, rotate the image so that the cranial aspect is on the left.

✓ To correlate the right lateral recumbent view to gross anatomy (Figure 2-2):

> Mentally picture the animal on its right side with the head to the left of your mental image.

> Mentally remove the left chest wall.

The difference between ventro-dorsal and dorso-ventral views are determined by the entry point of the x-ray beam to its exit point.

✓ Ventro-dorsal films are exposed with the patient in dorsal recumbency with the x-ray beam passing from ventral to dorsal.

✓ Dorso-ventral films are exposed with the patient in ventral recumbency with the x-ray beam passing from dorsal to ventral.

✓ By convention, ventro-dorsal/dorso-ventral views are placed on the view box with the right side to the viewer's left. The film is placed as though you could shake hands with your patient.

✓ To correlate the ventro-dorsal view to gross anatomy (Figure 2-3):

> Mentally picture the animal on its back with the right side on your left.

> Mentally remove the ventral body wall.

✓ To correlate the dorso-ventral view to gross anatomy (Figure 2-4):

> Mentally picture the animal on its sternum with the right side on your right.

> Mentally remove the dorsal structures.

> Using mental gymnastics, rotate the image so that right structures are on your left.

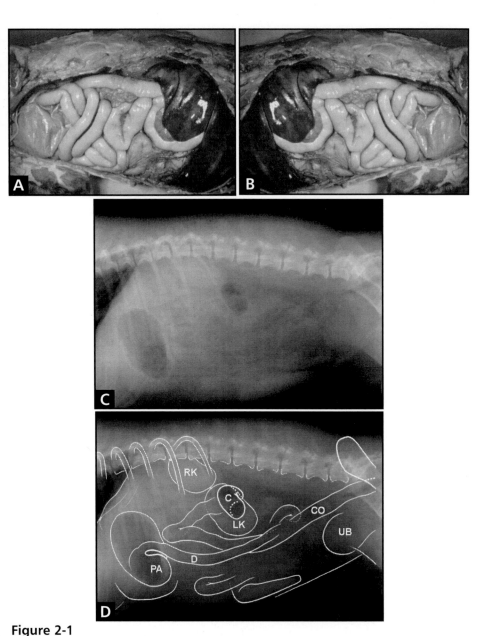

Figure 2-1
A. Gross image of a dog in left lateral recumbency with the right chest wall removed. **B.** Gross image rotated with "mental gymnastics" so that the head is to the left. **C.** Radiograph of a dog in left lateral recumbency. **D.** Diagram of a radiograph of a dog in left lateral recumbency shows major organs. RK: right kidney; C:cecum; LK:left kidney; PA:pyloric antrum; D:duodenum; CO:colon; UB:urinary bladder.

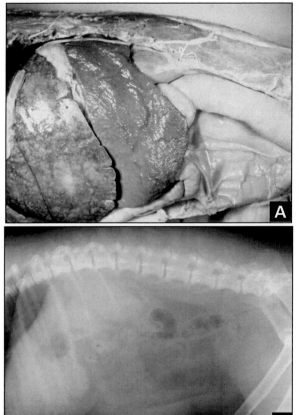

Figure 2-2
A. Gross image of a dog in right lateral recumbency with the left chest wall removed. **B.** Radiograph of a dog in right lateral recumbency. **C.** Diagram of a radiograph of a dog in right lateral recumbency shows major organs. RK: right kidney; LK:left kidney; C:cecum; CO:colon; D:duodenum; PA:pyloric antrum; SpT: tail of spleen.

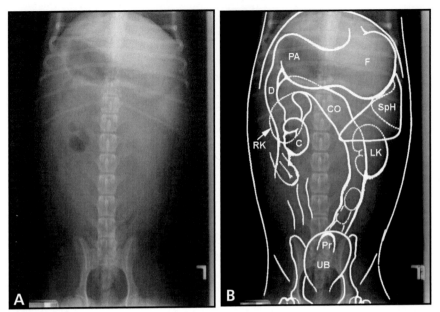

Figure 2-3
A. Ventro-dorsal view of the abdomen of a dog in dorsal recumbency.
B. Diagram of a ventro-dorsal radiograph of a dog in dorsal recumbency shows major organs.

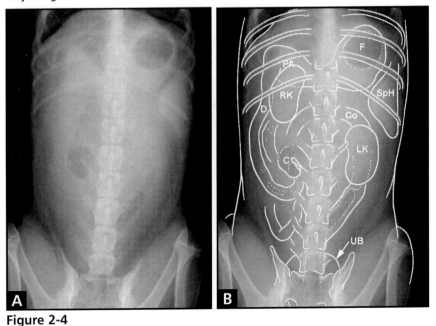

Figure 2-4
A. Dorsoventral view of the abdomen of a dog in ventral recumbency.
B. Diagram of a dorsoventral radiograph of a dog in ventral recumbency shows major organs.

15

Stomach

Dog

Lateral View

✓ The stomach is caudal to the liver.

♥ The long axis is at right angles to the spine, parallel to the ribs, or in-between.

✓ Pyloric antrum is cranial to or superimposed over the body of the stomach.

☠ If the left side is down, the pylorus (on the right side) will be "up" and air will move to fill the pylorus (see Figure 2-1).

> ✓ The diaphragm will have a v-shaped appearance in left lateral recumbency.

☠ If the right side is down, the pylorus will be "down" and it will be fluid-filled and may resemble a round ball (see Figure 2-2).

> 💣 Don't make the mistake of operating to remove a non-existent ball in the pylorus!!
>
> ✓ The diaphragm will have the appearance of two parallel lines (Figure 3-1) in right lateral recumbency.

Ventrodorsal/Dorsoventral View

✓ The stomach lies perpendicular to the spine across the abdomen with the pylorus near the right body wall.

✓ In some dogs, it may be u-shaped with a more obvious angular notch.

☠ If the dog is in dorsal recumbency (ventrodorsal view), the gastric body will be "up" and gas will move to the body (see Figure 2-3).

☠ If the dog is in ventral recumbency (dorsoventral view), the the fundus will be "up" and gas will fill the fundus (see Figure 2-4).

Cat

Lateral View

✓ The normal gastric axis is 30° caudal to a line perpendicular to the spine.

♥ Most cats have a large falciform fat pad elevating the liver and stomach.

Ventrodorsal/Dorsoventral View
♥ J-shaped stomach
✓ Pylorus is superimposed on or immediately to the right of the spine

Duodenum

✓ Dog: Pyloric antrum runs cranially to the cranial duodenal flexure; the descending duodenum runs caudally to the caudal flexure to become the ascending duodenum (Figure 2-5).

Cecum

✓ Located at L2-L4
♥ The cecum is shaped like a pig's tail in dogs (Figure 2-6)
♥ The cecum is small and comma-shaped in cats

Kidney

✓ Proper preparation of the abdomen (cleansing of the colon) is important for visualization of the kidneys.

Dog

✓ Fat in the retroperitoneal space allows the kidneys to be seen.

☗ The right kidney is cranial to the left and is located at the level of the 13th rib.

♥ The cranial pole of the right kidney is buried in the caudate process of the caudate lobe of the liver and is poorly seen.

♥ Lateral view: The caudal pole of the right kidney and the cranial pole of the left kidney are superimposed resulting in the appearance of a circular opacity (see Figures 2-1 and 2-2).

♠* In obese dogs, a large amount of fat in the retroperitoneal space causes the kidneys to be located in the midabdomen.

✓ Ventro-dorsal view: The right kidney is bisected by the right 13th rib (see Figures 2-3 and 2-4). The left kidney is located more caudally.

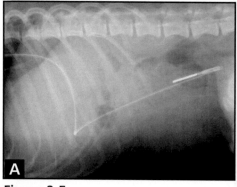

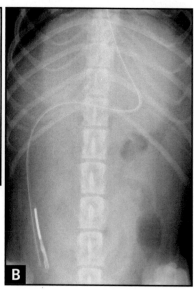

Figure 2-5
A. Lateral view of a dog shows a feeding tube in the esophagus, stomach, and duodenum. **B.** Ventrodorsal view of a dog shows a feeding tube in the esophagus, stomach, and duodenum.

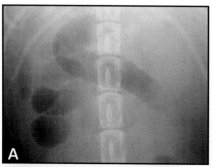

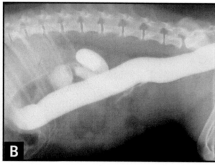

Figure 2-6
A. Normal gas-filled cecum in a dog.
B. Lateral barium enema in a dog shows the cecum. **C.** Ventrodorsal barium enema of the dog in Figure 2-6B. CC: cecocolic valve; IC: ileocolic valve; Tip: tip of the cecum.

Cat

✓ The kidneys are more mobile.

✓ The right kidney is more caudal and the cranial pole is visible (see Figures 1-1 and 2-7).

Length: Ventrodorsal view

Dog: 2.5-3.5 x L2

Cat: 2.4-3.0 x L2

Width: Ventrodorsal view

Dog: 2 +/-.2 x L2

Cat: 3.0-3.5 cm

Spleen

Dog

Lateral

✓ Splenic tail moves freely between L2-L4 and may cross the midline of the abdominal floor.

♥ The tail is seen as a rounded, somewhat triangular opacity on the abdominal floor (see Figures 2-1 and 2-2).

✓ The tail is best seen in the right lateral recumbent view as it crosses from left to right.

✓ The body of the spleen lies flat and is less likely to be seen.

✓ The head is sometimes seen as a triangular opacity cranial to the left kidney.

Ventrodorsal/Dorsoventral

♥ The head of the spleen appears as a triangle between the lateral aspects of the fundus and cranial pole of the left kidney, adjacent to the lateral body wall (see Figures 2-3 and 2-4). The head is relatively immobile as it is held in place by the gastrosplenic ligament.

Cat

✓ The feline spleen has a similar appearance to the dog's but it is usually smaller and less visible (Figure 2-7)

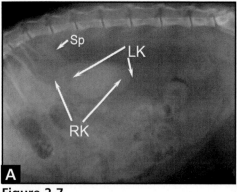
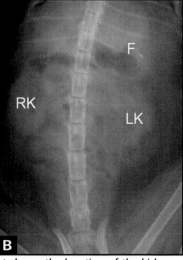

Figure 2-7
A. Lateral view of a cat shows the location of the kidneys. Notice that the proximal head of the spleen is visible cranial to the left kidney. The spleen is too small for the distal extremity or tail to be visible. **B.** Ventrodorsal view of a cat shows the location of the kidneys. Superimposition of fecal material in the colon interferes with visualization of the kidneys. Proper preparation of the abdomen is important! RK: right kidney; LK: left kidney; Sp: spleen; F: fundus.

Diaphragm

☗⊐ The liver and diaphragm are both fluid opaque (see Figures 2-1, 2-2, 2-3, and 2-4).

♥ In a normal abdomen, the liver and diaphragm blend together.

💣※ If air is present between the liver and diaphragm, the diaphragm shows as a fluid-opaque line cranial to the liver (Figure 2-8).

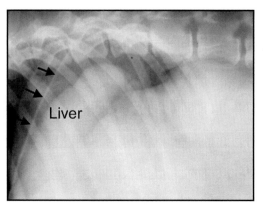

Figure 2-8
Lateral view of the abdomen of a dog shows air between the liver and diaphragm.

Liver

✓ The liver appears as a fluid opacity cranial to the stomach.

✓ Naturally occurring gastric gas can help identify the caudal hepatic border and aid in the assessment of liver size.

✓ Barium can be placed in the stomach to aid in differentiating liver and stomach (see page 46).

Lateral

✓ The ventral lobe margins should appear sharp.

✓ The caudal-ventral border is formed by the left lateral lobe.

Ventrodorsal/dorsoventral

✓ Cranial border of the right kidney is buried in the caudate lobe.

✓ Cranial duodenal flexure and fundus contact the right and left lateral lobes.

✓ Medial and quadrate lobes are adjacent to the lesser gastric curvature.

Bladder

✓ The urinary bladder is an oval structure in the ventral caudal abdomen.

✓ It can be seen because of the fat in the ventral and lateral ligaments, the omentum, and mesentery.

✓ In the dog, the neck of the bladder is near the pubis (see Figures 2-1 and 2-2).

✓ In the cat, the neck of the bladder is longer so that the bladder is located more cranially (see Figure 2-7).

Prostate

✓ The prostate gland is located at the neck of the urinary bladder.

✓ The urethra runs through the center of the prostate gland.

✓ In young or castrated dogs, the prostate gland may be intrapelvic and therefore may not be visible.

♥ In older dogs, the prostate is variably sized, and it will appear as a fluid opacity located just cranial to the pelvic brim (Figure 2-9A).

💣※ In the ventrodorsal view, remember to look for the prostate cranial to the pelvic brim and not cranial to the ilial wings (Figures 2-9B and 2-9C).

♥ The prostate gland is not visible in cats (same location but smaller).

Lymph Nodes

✓ The medial iliac lymph node is ventral to L6-7.

♥ The medial iliac lymph node is poorly visualized unless it is enlarged (Figure 2-10).

♥ Mesenteric and other visceral lymph nodes are not normally radiographically apparent.

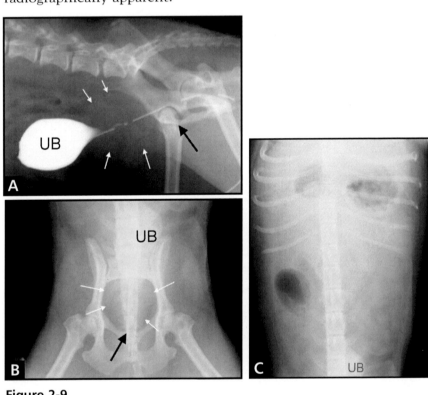

Figure 2-9
Male dog with moderate prostatic enlargement shows the relationship of the prostate gland (white arrows) to the pelvic brim (black arrow) and ilial wings **A.** Lateral view. Contrast is present in the urinary bladder (UB). **B.** Ventrodorsal view. **C.** This ventrodorsal view was exposed too far cranially for the prostate to be seen.

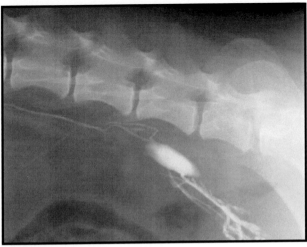

Figure 2-10
Lateral view of the dorsocaudal abdomen of a dog show-ing the medial iliac lymph node. Iodine contrast has been injected into the lymphatic system to show the location of the node which is normally not clearly seen.

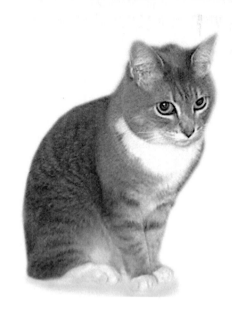

Section 3

Peritoneal Cavity

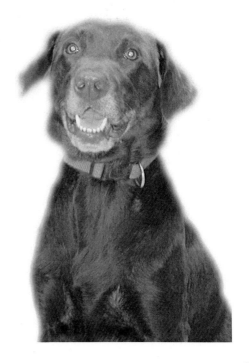

Normal Appearance

✓ Normal peritoneal cavity contains a small amount of fluid.

✓ Normal peritoneal fluid is not radiographically apparent.

☞ Serosal detail is visible because of the fat surrounding serosal surfaces (Figure 3-1).

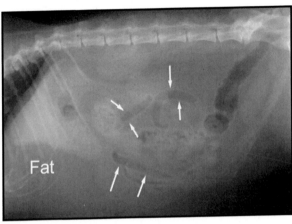

Figure 3-1
Very fat cat shows excellent serosal detail. Arrows point to serosal surfaces.

Increased Peritoneal Opacity

✓ Increased opacity can be regional or generalized.

✓ Increased opacity results in a loss of serosal detail that can be partial or complete.

☞ The key sign for an increased peritoneal opacity is failure or difficulty in visualizing serosal borders.

Terminology–Synonyms

✓ Loss of serosal detail

   Fluid opaque abdomen (total loss of serosal detail)

   Decreased or no visualization of serosal surfaces

   Increased intra-abdominal fluid (soft tissue) opacity

   Loss of intra-abdominal contrast

General Causes of a Loss of Serosal Detail

♥ Loss of fat for contrast

♥ Gain of fluid opacity that obscures fat

♥ Compression by mass

Specific Causes of a Loss of Serosal Detail

1. Young animal less than 3 months old (Figure 3-2) ⊙

2. Emaciation (loss of mesenteric fat). The abdomen may be "tucked up" or appear obviously thin (Figure 3-3) ⊙.

3. Peritoneal fluid – ascites, hemorrhage, chyle. Can confirm with paracentesis or diagnostic peritoneal lavage.

4. Peritonitis – edema and inflammation of serosal surfaces +/- effusion (Figure 3-4) ⊙

5. Rupture of a hollow organ- bile, urine, ingesta, purulent material (abscess, pyometra, Figure 3-5)

6. Peritoneal seeding with neoplastic foci ("carcinomatosis" can refer to seeding with carcinoma or other neoplasms).

7. Postoperative abdomen (1-2 weeks are required for absorption of serum, blood, and lymph).

8. Compression of organs by a mass.

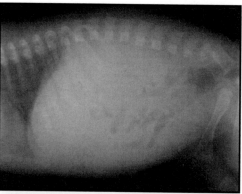

Figure 3-2
Lateral view of a 3-week old puppy shows a lack of serosal detail.

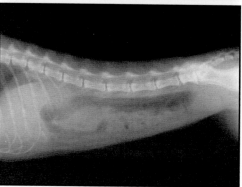

Figure 3-3
Lateral view of an emaciated cat (secondary to sublingual squamous cell carcinoma) shows a total loss of serosal detail (fluid opaque abdomen).

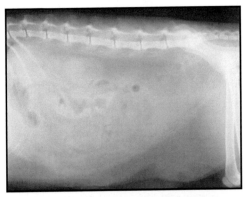

Figure 3-4
Lateral view of the abdomen of a dog with peritonitis shows a loss of serosal detail.

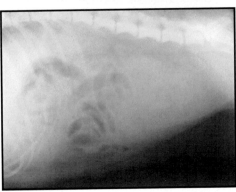

Figure 3-5
Lateral view of the abdomen of a dog with a ruptured uterus secondary to pyometra.

Radiographic (Roentgen) Signs

✓ The abdomen may appear "tucked up" in emaciation.

✓ The abdomen may be distended when fluid or a mass is present.

☞ If the abdomen is fluid opaque, mucosal surfaces may be visible but serosal surfaces are not seen.

💣 Remember that a fluid opaque abdomen can result from causes other than fluid in the abdomen.

✓ When fluid is present, the type of fluid cannot be distinguished radiographically. Paracentesis should be performed to determine what type of fluid is in the abdomen.

✓ In a partial loss of serosal detail, serosal surfaces can be seen but only with difficulty.

✓ The retroperitoneal space can be used for comparison.

Decreased Peritoneal Opacity–Gas

Distinguish between intraluminal and extraluminal gas accumulation.

Causes of Intraluminal Gas Accumulation

✓ Normal: fundus, duodenum, caecum, colon

✓ Aerophagia-dyspnea, struggle, anesthesia

✓ Ileus, functional

✓ Ileus, mechanical (obstruction)

Causes of Extraluminal Gas Accumulation

✓ Abdominal surgery-gas persists after abdominal surgery for days to weeks.

✓ Paracentesis

✓ Gas-forming organisms

✓ Ruptured hollow organ (e.g., perforated ulcer, gun shot causing ruptured GI tract)

💣※ Visualization of free abdominal gas can represent an emergency medical condition.

✓ Consider the possibility of a ruptured hollow organ.

✓ Emergency exploratory surgery may be indicated.

Radiographic (Roentgen) Signs of Extraluminal Gas

1. Larger Amounts (Figures 2-8 and 3-6) ⊙

    ♥ May see gas between diaphragm and liver; holding the dog on his hind legs for 5 minutes before taking the radiograph will improve the chance of seeing that gas.

    ♥ Look for sharp-edged gas shapes (i.e., triangles, etc) rather than the rounded shapes (ovals, circles) that are seen with intraluminal gas.

    ✓ Serosal surfaces will seem brighter and more obvious because of increased contrast.

✔ Air-fluid interface can be seen if the abdomen is exposed with a horizontal beam and both air and fluid are present.

✔ Small bubbles may be seen in the mesentery, spleen, or other tissues.

2. Small Amounts

✔ Use a horizontal beam with the animal in left lateral recumbency (fundus down).

✔ Free peritoneal gas is seen between liver and peritoneum (Figure 3-7). ⊙

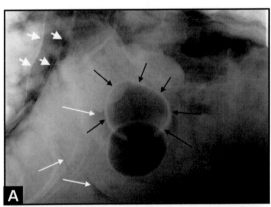

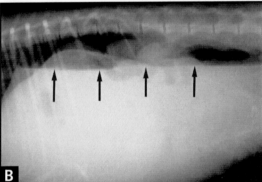

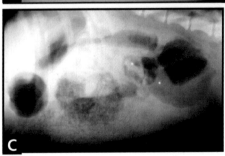

Figure 3-6
A. Lateral view of the abdomen of a German Shepherd dog with intra-abdominal gas secondary to multifocal neoplasia. The dog also had pneumothorax and pneumomediastinum. Note the sharp edged geometric shapes (long white arrows) rather than circles or ovals and the bright serosal surfaces (long black arrows). Gas is between the liver and the dorsal halves of the diaphragm (short white arrows). **B.** Lateral view of a dog with a gastric rupture. The film was exposed with the dog in lateral recumbency using a horizontal beam. An air-fluid interface (arrows) is seen. **C.** Lateral view of the abdomen of a dog with splenic torsion shows loculated gas bubbles in the spleen secondary to splenic necrosis.

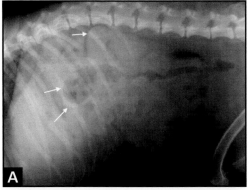

Figure 3-7
A. Lateral view of a dog hit by a car 3 days prior. Serosal surfaces are more visible than usual (arrows). **B.** A film was exposed using a horizontal beam with the dog in right lateral recumbency (although left lateral recumbency is preferred to avoid confusion with the gastric fundus). F: gastric fundus. G: gas between the liver and abdominal wall.

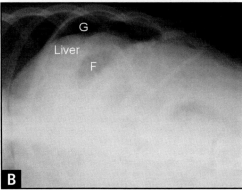

Decreased Peritoneal Opacity–Fat

Causes of Abnormal Fat Opacities
✓ Obesity

✓ Neoplasms (lipoma, liposarcoma)

Radiographic (Roentgen) Signs
✓ Abnormal fat accumulations will be seen as an area of decreased opacity (Figure 3-8).

✓ Remember that fat is more radiopaque than gas but less radiopaque than fluid.

✓ Fat may be unusually distributed.

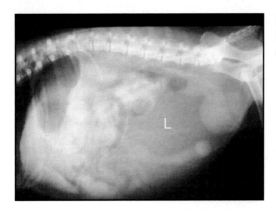

Figure 3-8
Lateral view of the abdomen of a dog with a liposarcoma.

Disruption of Borders of the Peritoneal Cavity

✓ Herniation of abdominal organs through the diaphragm, abdominal wall, or perineal tissues.

✓ Ultrasonography can be useful to identify displaced organs.

Diaphragmatic Hernia

"Ruptured" diaphragm (Figures 3-9A and 3-9B)

✓ A hernia's appearance varies depending on which organs pass through the tear.

✓ Herniated contents can include liver, spleen, stomach, intestines, and omentum.

Roentgen Signs on Survey Radiography

✓ Diaphragmatic shadow is interrupted.

✓ Pleural effusion can be present.

✓ Circular or oval air opacities in thorax may indicate gas within displaced GI tract.

✓ Herniated solid organs (liver, spleen) can present as a solid fluid opacity in the thorax

Roentgen Signs on Contrast Radiography

➤ Purpose is to put contrast into or around a herniated organ

Upper GI series will help if portions of the GI tract are herniated (Figure 3-9C)

✓ You could conceivably put iodine contrast in vessels (arteriography), although it would be impractical

✓ Celiography can be diagnostic

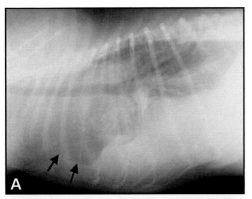

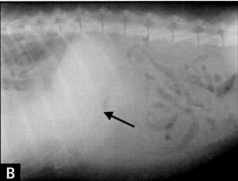

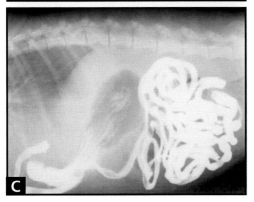

Figure 3-9
A. Lateral view of the thorax of a dog with a diaphragmatic hernia shows disruption of the diaphragm. Pleural effusion is present causing retraction of the edges of the lung lobes (black arrows). **B.** Lateral view of the abdomen of a dog with a diaphragmatic hernia shows displacement of the stomach. Air is present in the lumen of the stomach. **C.** Barium contrast aids in identification of the stomach.

Celiography

☞ Inject 350 to 400 milligrams/kilograms of sterile organic iodide solution into the peritoneal cavity (Figure 3-10) ⊙

✓ Inject the iodide solution with the animal in dorsal recumbency at the level of the umbilicus.

✓ The main indication is confirmation of abdominal hernias

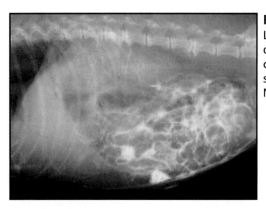

Figure 3-10
Lateral celiogram of a normal dog 5 minutes after injection of contrast. Iodine contrast can be seen between serosal surfaces. No contrast is in the thorax.

Hiatal Hernia

✓ Hernia of stomach: stomach with or without gastroesoplageal sphincter through the esophageal hiatus (Figure 3-11)

✓ Sliding hiatal hernia: gastroesophageal sphincter and part of the stomach move in and out of the thorax.

✓ Paraesophageal hiatal hernia: part of the stomach remains alongside the esophagus.

Roentgen Signs on Survey Films

✓ Fluid +/- air opacity in the region of the caudal esophagus in thoracic film

Roentgen Signs on Contrast Study

✓ Barium or water soluble iodine contrast is given orally in order to identify the stomach.

✓ To diagnose sliding hernias, you may have to elevate the animal's hind end.

Peritoneopericardial Hernia

Abdominal organs herniate through a congenital defect into the pericardial sac (Figure 3-12). This kind of hernia may be an incidental finding or it may cause clinical signs.

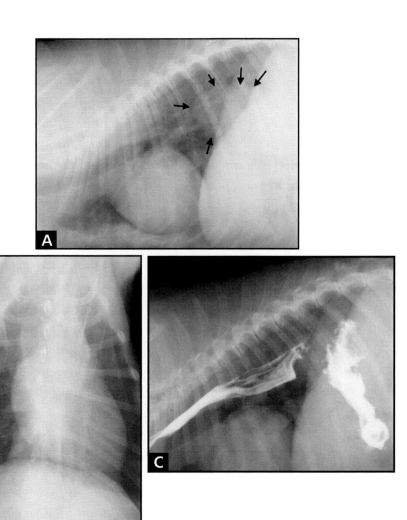

Figure 3-11
A. Lateral view of the thorax of a mixed-breed dog with a sliding hiatal hernia. Black arrows indicate a fluid opacity seen in the caudo-dorsal lung field on survey radiography of the thorax. **B.** When the dog was positioned for a ventrodorsal radiograph, the opacity disappeared. **C.** An esophagram performed during fluoroscopy confirmed that the opacity was the stomach sliding in and out of the esophagus.

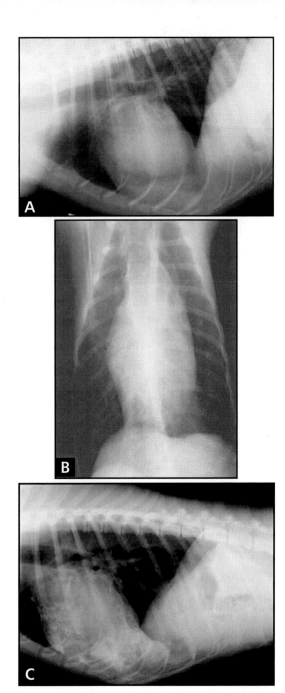

Figure 3-12

A 2-year old spayed Border Collie with exercise intolerance. **A.** Lateral view of the thorax shows an unusual fat/fluid opacity ventral to the heart. **B.** Ventrodorsal view. **C.** A radiograph exposed 15 minutes after the injection of water soluble iodine contrast into the abdomen (celiography) shows a peritoneopericardial hernia.

Roentgen Signs on Survey Films

✓ Gas may be seen in bowel loops superimposed over the heart shadow.

✓ Cardiac silhouette may appear larger than normal.

✓ In the lateral view, the ventral cardiac silhouette blends with the diaphragm/liver.

✓ In the ventrodorsal view, the cardiac silhouette blends with the diaphragm/liver.

Roentgen Signs on Contrast Study

✓ In an upper GI, oral barium can be given to identify the stomach and small intestine.

♥ In celiography, iodine contrast will flow cranially from the peritoneal cavity into the pericardial sac.

Inguinal or Ventral Hernias

✓ Muscle tearing that is often associated with trauma leads to hernias through the abdominal wall or inguinal ring.

Roentgen Signs on Survey Films

♥ A loss of integrity can occur in the abdominal wall (Figures 3-13 and 3-14).

✓ Soft tissue swelling at the herniation site

✓ Gas-filled loops of intestine might be seen outside the peritoneal cavity.

✓ An inability to identify the urinary bladder could indicate that it is displaced.

Roentgen Signs on Contrast Study

✓ Cystography can be used to identify the urinary bladder (Figure 3-13).

✓ Upper GI series with oral barium could be performed to identify displaced bowel loops.

✓ Celiography might confirm tearing of the abdominal wall (Figure 3-14). ◉

Perineal Hernia

✓ Tearing of the perineal tissues often occurs secondary to trauma

Roentgen Signs on Survey Films

✓ Abnormal soft tissue swelling is seen in the perineal region.

✓ Loss of visualization of the prostate or bladder could indicate displacement of these organs.

✓ Fecal material or ingesta can be seen in displaced bowel loops.

Roentgen Signs on Contrast Study

✓ Urethrography, cystography, upper GI series, and a barium enema can be used to identify displaced organs (Figure 3-15). ◉

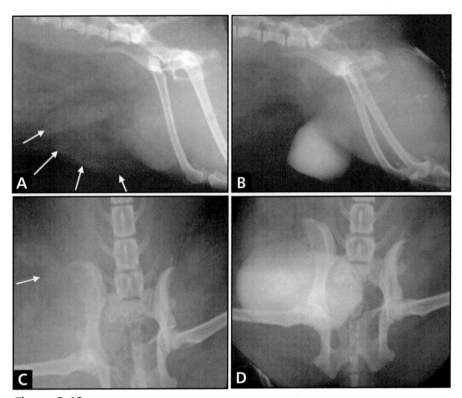

Figure 3-13
A. Lateral view of a 4-year old Chihuahua that had a fractured pelvis after being hit by a car. Arrows indicate an inguinal hernia. **B.** Lateral view of a cystogram shows the urinary bladder in the hernial sac. **C.** Ventrodorsal view shows the fractured pelvis and inguinal hernia on the right side. The white arrow shows the point of disruption of the abdominal wall. **D.** Ventrodorsal view of a cystogram shows the urinary bladder in the hernial sac.

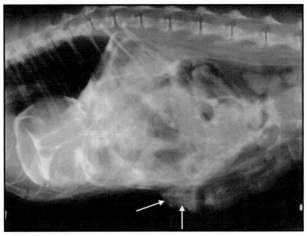

Figure 3-14
Radiograph of a 12-year old Persian cat presented with pleural effusion. Survey radiographs suggested a possible diaphragmatic hernia. Additionally, numerous ventral hernias could be palpated. Celiography showed that the diaphragm was intact but bulging (no contrast is seen in the thorax). Contrast enhances visualization of the ventral hernias (arrows).

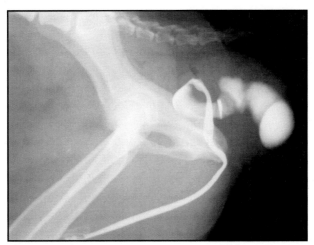

Figure 3-15
Radiograph of an Irish Setter with a perineal hernia. A lateral urethrogram shows the urinary bladder displaced caudally.

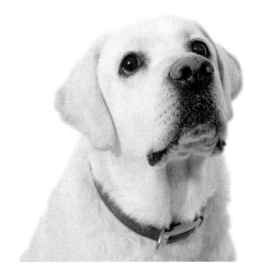

Intra-abdominal Masses

Evaluation of an Abdominal Mass

✓ The study of possible masses is an excellent way to learn radiographic anatomy.

✓ Describe the mass in terms of size, shape, position, opacity, and margination of the mass.

✓ Evaluate displacement of other organs.

✓ Consider the mobility of organs that are suspected to be involved in the mass.

Gastric Masses

Roentgen Signs

The cranial mass is caudal to the liver.

The small intestine, transverse colon, and spleen will be pushed caudad.

During gastric torsion, the spleen may be enlarged due to congestion or torsion.

Examples of Gastric Masses

✓ Full stomach (Figure 4-1)

✓ Neoplasia (Figure 4-2) ⊙

✓ Adenocarcinoma is most common in dogs; lymphosarcoma is most common in cats.

💣※ It can be difficult to distinguish between the liver and the stomach.

Generalized Hepatomegaly

Roentgen Signs

Cranial mass

  Lateral view (Figure 4-3A)

- ✓ The normal gastric axis will be pushed dorso-caudally.
- ✓ Ventral liver margins may be rounded.
- ✓ The pyloric antrum will be located more dorsal and caudal.

Ventro-dorsal view (Figure 4-3B)

- ✓ The gastric body and pyloric antrum will be pushed caudally.

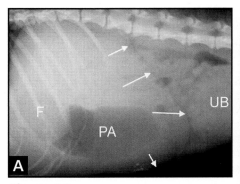

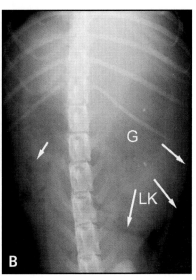

Figure 4-1
Radiograph of a dog with a fluid-filled stomach secondary to a foreign body (F) at the pylorus. Arrows indicate the caudal margins of the stomach. PA: pyloric antrum; G: gas bubble in the stomach; UB: urinary bladder; LK: left kidney. **A.** Lateral view. **B.** Ventrodorsal view.

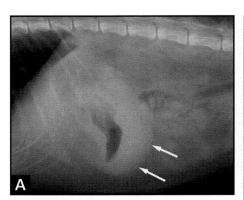

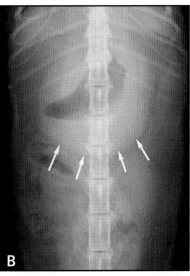

Figure 4-2
Gastric lymphosarcoma in a cat. Arrows indicate the caudal margin of the stomach. **A.** Lateral view. **B.** Ventrodorsal view. Ultrasound-guided aspiration confirmed lymphosarcoma.

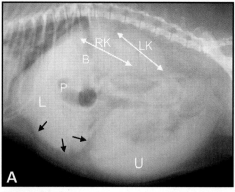
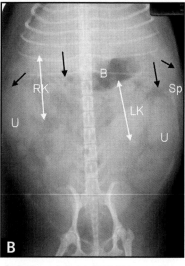

Figure 4-3
Generalized liver enlargement in an 8.5-year old female Poodle with liver disease and pyometra. The uterus (U) is enlarged. Liver enlargement pushed the gastric body (B) caudally. Double-headed arrows indicate the left (LK) and right (RK) kidneys (the cranial pole of the right kidney is buried in the caudate process of the liver and is not clearly seen). P: location of the pyloric valve; Sp: spleen. **A.** Lateral view. **B.** Ventrodorsal view.

Focal Hepatomegaly

A) Right lateral and right medial

✓ Focal hepatomegaly affects structures on the right side such as the pyloric antrum, pylorus, proximal descending duodenum, ascending colon, and the adjacent small intestine (Figure 4-4).

✓ Right-sided structures are pushed caudally, dorsally, and medially.

✓ Some hepatic masses are pedunculated, and a portion can become located caudal to the stomach by pushing the gastric body cranially and dorsally.

B) Left lateral and left medial

✓ Affects structures on the left side such as the splenic head, adjacent small intestine, and gastric fundus.

✓ Affected structures are pushed dorsally and medially.

✓ The splenic tail is pushed to variable locations.

✓ A pedunculated mass may push the gastric fundus cranially and dorsally.

C) Central

✓ Central structures are affected such as the gastric body and adjacent small intestine.

✓ The affected structures are pushed caudally and dorsally.

✓ The serosal border of the lesser curvature may be indented.

Differentiate the Stomach

✓ Differentiating between hepatic and splenic masses can be difficult.

♥ Opposite views may help by shifting the location of the gastric gas bubble.

♥ Contrast can be placed within the gastric lumen (Figure 4-5). ⊙

✓ Ultrasound can be useful.

Remember the flip side! Microhepatica (See page 152).

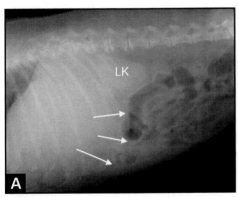

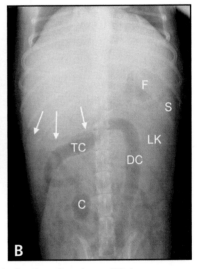

Figure 4-4
A 10-year old Shetland Sheepdog with a focal right-sided liver enlargement. Arrows indicate the caudal margin of the liver. Notice the similarity of the enlarged liver to an enlarged stomach. LK: left kidney, F: gastric fundus, S: spleen, TC: transverse colon, DC: descending colon, C: cecum. **A.** Lateral view. **B.** Ventrodorsal view.

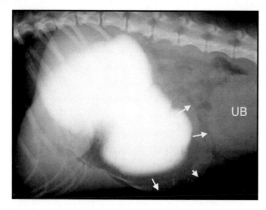

Figure 4-5
Lateral view of the abdomen of the dog in Figure 4-1. Barium was put in the stomach to confirm that the mass was an enlarged stomach. Arrows indicate the caudal margins of the stomach. UB:urinary bladder.

Renal Masses

Roentgen Signs

✓ The kidneys are firmly fastened in the dorsal retroperitoneal space.

☛ Renal masses stay dorsal!

💣 It may not be obvious that large masses originated dorsally unless both views are evaluated (Figure 4-6).

✓ Most other retroperitoneal masses permit visualization of the kidneys; adrenal gland masses may be an exception.

A) Right kidney

✓ The caudal pole is not visible as a structure separate from the mass (normally you will only see the caudal pole).

✓ Affected structures are on the right, including the descending duodenum, ascending colon, and the adjacent small intestine.

✓ Affected structures are pushed ventrally and to the left.

B) Left kidney

✓ The left kidney is not seen separately from the mass. Usually you can see all of the left kidney.

✓ Affected structures are on the left, such as the descending colon and adjacent small intestine.

✓ Affected structures are pushed ventrally and to the right.

✓ Contrast examination of the kidneys is useful to confirm a renal mass.

✓ Contrast examination can also help identify a perirenal pseudocyst (see page 133).

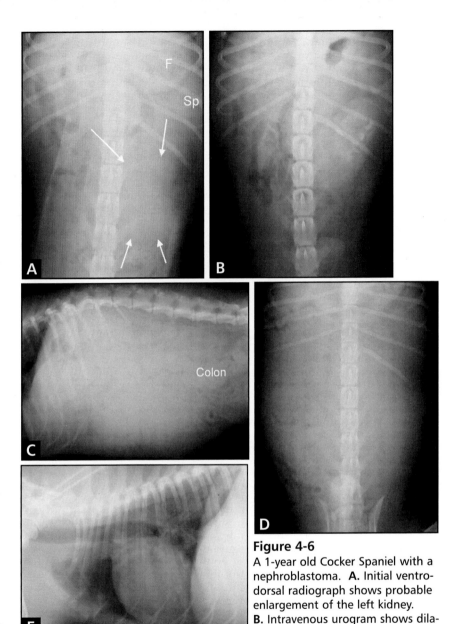

Figure 4-6
A 1-year old Cocker Spaniel with a nephroblastoma. **A.** Initial ventro-dorsal radiograph shows probable enlargement of the left kidney. **B.** Intravenous urogram shows dilation of the renal pelvis. **C.** In a lateral radiograph, made 1 month after initial presentation, there appears to be a ventral mass. **D.** The ventrodorsal view made 1 month after initial presentation shows that the mass (LK) occupies the left side of the abdomen from dorsal to ventral displacing small intestine (SI) and colon (C) to the right. Reexamination of the lateral view shows that the apparent dorsal edge of the mass is actually associated with the wall of the colon. **E.** Lateral thoracic radiograph shows the presence of metastatic nodules. (Initial radiographs are courtesy of Dr. Martha Thomas, North Gay Street Veterinary Clinic, Auburn, AL.)

47

Adrenal Mass

♥ Normal adrenal glands are not visible radiographically.

✓ Most adrenal masses are too small to be visible radiographically.

Roentgen Signs

✓ Mineralization of the adrenal glands could be associated with a neoplasm or with Cushing's disease, or it may be incidental.

✓ Adrenal glands are soft tissue and are fluid opaque, so the border between an enlarged adrenal gland and the adjacent kidney may not be visible.

✓ Occasionally, the adrenal gland can present as a distinct mass, located dorsally cranio-medial to the ipsilateral kidney (Figure 4-7).⊙

✓ A large mass might appear as a dorsal midabdominal mass.

Diffuse Splenomegaly

✓ Diffuse splenomegaly occurs with conditions such as congestion and torsion.

✓ Splenic torsion can occur +/- gastric torsion (Figure 4-8).⊙

Roentgen Signs

✓ Margins of the spleen are rounded.

✓ Adjacent organs are pushed away from the mass.

✓ With torsion, the spleen will be displaced and gas may be present.

Focal Splenomegaly

Roentgen Signs

A) Proximal extremity (head)

♥ Located on the left, fixed in place against the gastric fundus by the gastrosplenic ligament.

Lateral View

✓ Adjacent small intestine is pushed caudo-dorsally.

✓ Gastric fundus may be indented.

Ventrodorsal View

✓ The small intestine is pushed caudally and to the right.

✓ Gastric fundus may be indented.

B) Body/distal extremity

✓ Ventral or midabdominal mass (Figure 4-9) ⊙

Lateral View

✓ Mass caudal to the stomach located ventrally or midway between the spine and abdominal floor.

✓ The small intestine is pushed dorsally and cranially and/or caudally.

Ventrodorsal View

✓ The small intestine is pushed either to the left or right depending on the size of the spleen and location of the mass.

💣※ Small masses will not be radiographically apparent.

🔑 Splenic masses are the most common midabdominal or ventral midabdominal masses.

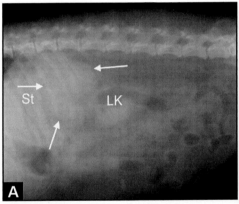
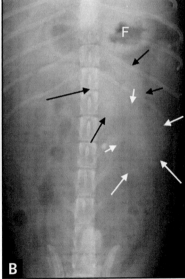

Figure 4-7
A. Lateral view of the abdomen of a 10-year old dog with an adrenal mass. Arrows indicate the mass, which is pushing the stomach cranially and the left kidney caudo-ventrally. St:stomach; LK:left kidney.
B. Ventrodorsal view shows the adrenal mass cranio-medially to the left kidney. F:fundus: white arrows, left kidney; black arrows, adrenal mass.

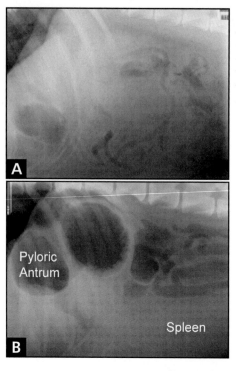

Figure 4-8
A. Lateral view of the abdomen of a dog with splenic torsion without gastric torsion. **B.** Lateral view of the abdomen of a dog with splenic torsion and gastric torsion after decompression of the stomach.

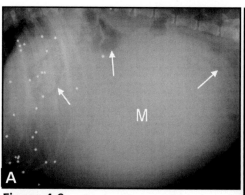
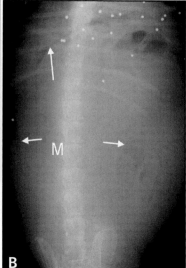

Figure 4-9
A 12-year old intact female Chow Chow with a large splenic mass (M). The small intestines (arrows) are pushed cranially, dorsally, and caudally. Notice the similarity in appearance to the enlarged mesenteric lymph node in Figure 4-11 and the pyometra in the tip of one horn in Figure 7-2. **A.** Lateral view. **B.** Ventrodorsal view.

Mesenteric/Enteric Masses

Roentgen Signs

A) Root of the mesentery

Lateral View (Figure 4-10)

✓ A poorly defined opacity appears in the midabdomen.

✓ The small intestine is pushed cranially, dorsally, and caudally.

✓ Rarely, one very large node may appear well-defined and resemble a splenic mass (Figure 4-11).

Ventrodorsal View

✓ The small intestine is pushed peripherally.

B) Elsewhere

✓ The small intestine will be pushed away from the mass.

C) Enteric mass (Figure 4-12)

✓ Neoplasia in the intestinal wall can become sufficiently large that a fluid opacity can be seen on survey radiographs.

Figure 4-10
Lateral view of the abdomen of a 6-year old dog with lymphosarcoma. Serosal detail is poor because of enlarged mesenteric lymph nodes. The sublumbar lymph nodes are also enlarged. M: root of the mesentery; SLLN:sublumbar lymph nodes; Sp:spleen.

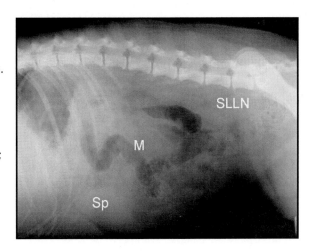

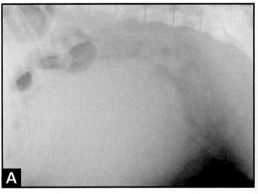

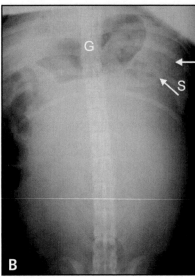

Figure 4-11

A 9-year old Boxer with a single enlarged mesenteric lymph node secondary to hemangiosarcoma. The spleen was normal at surgery but there was marked involvement of the mesenteric vessels. **A.** Lateral view. The mass pushes the intestines cranially, dorsally, and caudally. **B.** Ventrodorsal view. The mass occupies most of the abdomen. Arrows indicate the margins of the gastric fundus. G:Gas in the gastric lumen; S:spleen.

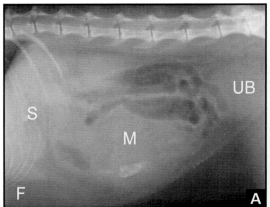

Figure 4-12

A 20-year old cat with an intestinal mass. The mass contains some areas of mineralization and is located in the mid abdomen on the right side, displacing small intestines to the left. M:mass, F:falciform fat, UB:urinary bladder, S:stomach. **A.** Lateral view. **B.** Ventrodorsal view.

Pancreatic Masses

Roentgen Signs
✓ Contrast may be needed to localize the duodenum
✓ Gas may be in the duodenum.
✓ Serosal surfaces may be poorly defined, particularly if fluid is present (Figure 4-13). ⊙

A) Left limb
✓ Located along the greater curvature of the stomach.

  Lateral View
    ✓ Duodenum is pushed ventrally.

  Ventrodorsal View
    ✓ The descending duodenum is pushed to the right.
    ✓ The caudal right aspect of the pyloric antrum may be indented.

B) Right limb
✓ The right limb is located dorso-medial to the descending duodenum.
✓ Gastric wall is not indented.
✓ Gas may be in the duodenum, although it can also be present normally.

  Lateral View
    ✓ The adjacent descending duodenum is pushed ventrally.
    ✓ Fluid opacity may be present in the area of the pancreas.

  Ventrodorsal View
    ✓ Adjacent descending duodenum is pushed to the right.
    ✓ Ascending colon may be pushed caudally and medially.

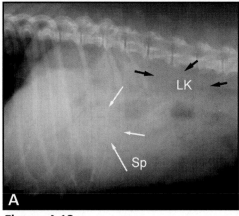
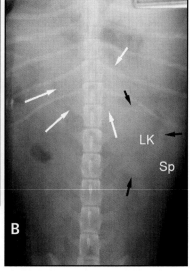

Figure 4-13
A 9-year old Chihuahua with a pancreatic mass confirmed during surgery as neoplasia. The mass (white arrows) is poorly defined but can be seen caudal to the stomach. The right kidney is not clearly seen. The left kidney (LK) is outlined by black arrows. Sp:spleen. **A.** Lateral view. **B.** Ventrodorsal view.

Ovarian Masses

Roentgen Signs

A) Right ovary

✓ Well defined homogeneous mass appears caudal to and separate from the right kidney (Figure 4-14).

♥ Ovarian ligaments stretch readily, so when the ovary enlarges, gravity sends it to the abdominal floor where it pushes the descending duodenum and ascending colon medially.

✓ A large mass can pull the caudal pole of the right kidney ventrally.

B) Left ovary

✓ A well-defined homogeneous mass appears caudal to and separate from the left kidney.

♥ When the ovary enlarges, the mass falls to the abdominal floor and pulls the descending colon and adjacent small intestine medially.

✓ A large mass can pull the caudal pole of the left kidney ventrally.

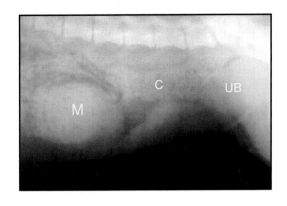

Figure 4-14
Lateral view of the abdomen of a dog shows a granulosa cell tumor in one ovary. M: ovarian mass, C:colon, UB:urinary bladder. Notice that the ovary falls to the floor of the abdomen.

Masses Involving Urinary Bladder

✓ Transitional cell carcinoma is the most common bladder neoplasm.

☞ Most neoplasms are not radiographically apparent without the use of contrast media.

✓ Most urinary bladder "masses" are overly distended urinary bladders (Figure 4-15).

✓ Most bladder tumors grow into the lumen and require cystography to be detected (See page 116).

Figure 4-15
Ventrodorsal view of a dog with a distended (but normal) urinary bladder (UB). The right (RK) and left (LK) kidneys can be faintly seen superimposed over the "mass". S:spleen.

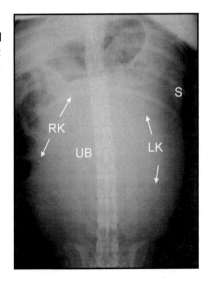

Roentgen Signs

✓ Mass in caudoventral abdomen

✓ Some bladder masses may have mineralization

Lateral View

✓ Small intestine is pushed cranially.

✓ Colon is pushed dorsally.

Ventrodorsal View

✓ Descending colon is pushed to the left or right

Prostatic Masses

Roentgen Signs

✓ The lateral view is the most useful.

✓ Remember to look for the prostate at the brim of the pelvis in the ventrodorsal view.

A) Symmetric enlargement

Lateral View (Figure 4-16) ⊙

✓ Urinary bladder is pushed cranially.

✓ +/- colon pushed dorsally

B) Asymmetric enlargement

Lateral View

✓ Urinary bladder is pushed cranio-ventrally or cranio-dorsally.

💣✳ **Tip!** An enlarged prostate can mimic the urinary bladder if the urinary bladder is empty (Figure 4-17).

✓ Both the prostate and urinary bladder are caudoventral structures.

Uterine Masses

♥ The uterus diameter must be greater than that of the small intestine for the uterus to be recognized.

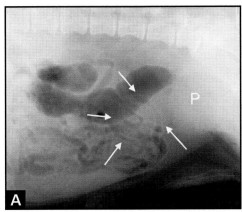

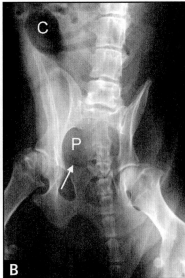

Figure 4-16
Radiographs of an 11-year old male Basset Hound with an enlarged prostate gland secondary to prostatic abscess. **A.** Lateral view. P:prostate, white arrows outline the urinary bladder. **B.** Ventrodorsal view. C:colon; P:prostate. Remember to look for the enlarged prostate immediately cranial to the pelvic brim (white arrow).

Figure 4-17
Lateral views of the abdomen of a 10-year old mixed-breed dog with a prostatic mass. The palpable prostatic mass does not appear to be visible in survey radiography. The presence of pulmonary nodules indicates pulmonary metastasis (white arrows). The medial iliac lymph nodes are enlarged and proliferative bone is along the ventral aspect of the spine. LK:left kidney; MI:medial iliac lymph nodes. **A.** Lateral survey radiograph. ?=bladder or prostate. **B.** Cystography identified the urinary bladder, which is normal. RK:right kidney; B:bladder; P: prostate. The urinary catheter is seen as a lucent band at the tip of the black arrow.

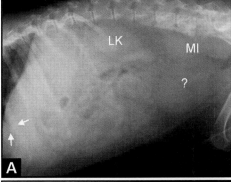

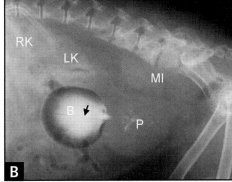

✔ The uterus is located in the caudoventral abdomen.

✔ Pyometra is the most common condition causing pathologic uterine enlargement.

●✳ Remember to keep normal pregnancy in the differential list.

Roentgen Signs

⌐ Tortuous tubular opacities are seen in the caudoventral abdomen (Figure 4-18).

Lateral View

> ✔ The small intestine is pushed dorsally and cranially.
>
> ✔ The colon and bladder will be separated more than usual.

Ventrodorsal View

> ✔ Tortuous horns are less easy to recognize with the ventrodorsal view than with the lateral view.
>
> ✔ The small intestine is pushed cranially and centrally.
>
> ✔ A wooden spoon or commercially available paddle can be used to move intestinal loops out of the way.

Caudal Sublumbar Masses

✔ These masses primarily involve the sublumbar lymph nodes, especially the medial iliac, and muscles.

✔ Consider neoplasia (primary lymphosarcoma or metastatic from the pelvic region), granulomas, and abscesses.

Roentgen Signs

Lateral View

> ♥ Broad-based homogeneous opacity in caudal sublumbar area (Figure 4-19).
>
> ✔ Descending colon may be displaced ventrally.
>
> ✔ Don't over read: the colon can travel ventrally without a mass being present.

Ventrodorsal View

> ✔ The lateral view is not very useful but some increased opacity might be seen lateral to the spine.

Remember to prioritize your differentials.

ALWAYS get thoracic radiographs to check for pulmonary metastasis!

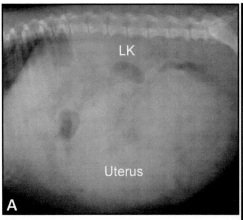

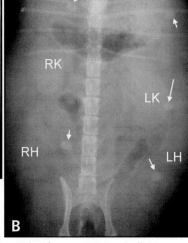

Figure 4-18
A 14-year old cat with pyometra shows markedly enlarged tortuous uterine horns in the ventral abdomen. LK:left kidney; RK:right kidney; RH:right uterine horn; LH:left uterine horn. Arrows indicate enlarged mammary nipples. **A.** Lateral view. **B.** Ventrodorsal view.

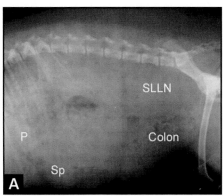

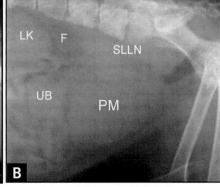

Figure 4-19
A. Lateral view of a castrated male Pomeranian with lymphosarcoma shows enlarged sublumbar lymph nodes (SLLN) pushing the colon ventrally. P: pylorus; Sp:spleen. Multiple enlarged mesenteric lymph nodes and a retained testicle are seen. **B.** Lateral view of the dog in Figure 4-17 shows a closer view of the retroperitoneal space. Notice the normal fat (F) in the retroperitoneal space separating the caudal pole of the left kidney (LK) and the enlarged sublumbar lymph nodes (SLLN). UB:urinary bladder; PM:prostate mass.

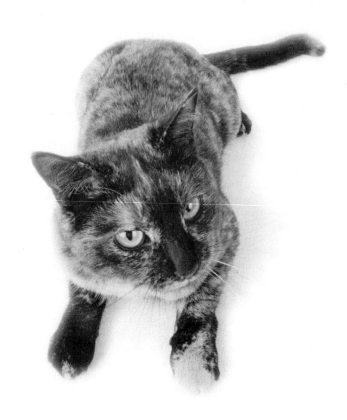

Section 5

Alimentary Tract

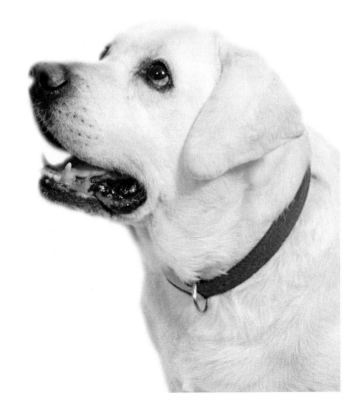

Contrast Media

✓ Contrast media is needed because of poor natural subject contrast in the abdomen.

✓ Materials are given to visualize organs or organ systems.

✓ Contrast media is commonly used to evaluate alimentary and urinary systems.

✓ Negative contrast media (less opaque contrast material)

Gases absorb few x-rays (radiolucent)

Appear black, e.g., air, carbon dioxide

✓ Positive contrast media (opaque contrast material)

Absorb a large portion of x-rays from the beam

Appear white, e.g., ionic iodine, non-ionic iodine, barium sulfate

✓ Double contrast procedures

Use both positive and negative contrast media

Barium

✓ Barium is less expensive than iodine.

♥ It provides excellent mucosal coating.

✓ Not absorbed or diluted

✓ Stays in suspension

✓ Cure? A common observation is that administration of oral barium often results in remission of clinical signs even when a diagnosis cannot be made.

But:

💣☀ Barium is harmful in the peritoneal cavity. **Do not use barium when you suspect a ruptured or lacerated GI tract.**

Barium causes a fulminating granulomatous inflammatory response in the peritoneal cavity.

✓ It creates an added complication if surgery is necessary, although its use does not preclude surgery.

✓ Problems can occur if a large volume of barium is inhaled, so make sure the stomach tube is properly placed!

✓ Slower transit than iodine media

Ionic Organic Iodine

✓ Ionic organic iodine is water soluble

✓ Innocuous in peritoneal cavity

✓ Rapid transit

But ionic organic iodine is

✓ Expensive

✓ It doesn't coat mucosa well.

✓ Hypertonicity causes fluid to enter the GI tract from the tissues, reducing radiopacity.

💣※ Hypertonicity can lead to dehydration or hypovolemic shock. **Do not use ionic organic iodine in dehydrated animals (vomiting, diarrhea)!**

✓ Irritating, and subsequent diarrhea can occur.

💣※ *Can cause pulmonary edema if inhaled. **Do not use ionic organic iodine if aspiration is likely.**

Non-Ionic Organic Iodine Preparations

✓ Non-ionic organic iodine (Iohexol, Iopamidol) has the advantages of ionic organic iodine and is NOT hypertonic; it does not cause the side effects associated with hypertonicity.

But:

✓ Newer and still MUCH MORE expensive

✓ It does not coat mucosa well (see page 104 for dosages).

Esophageal/Gastrointestinal Contrast Procedures

✓ Use esophageal/gastrointestinal contrast procedures when diagnosis or determination of the course of therapy cannot be made from the survey radiographs and other clinical information.

🔑 Always take survey radiographs immediately before contrast.

The survey radiograph might give the answer.

It provides a baseline.

An ultrasound may be an alternative or contributory.

Positive contrast media will not interfere with ultrasound examination.

Radiography of the Esophagus

Survey Radiographs

✓ The esophagus is not normally seen.

✓ Esophagus is a fluid-opaque structure blending with other fluid opaque structures in the cervical area or mediastinum. A vague radiopacity may be seen in the caudodorsal thorax in the lateral view.

✓ Air does not normally stay in the esophagus.

✓ A small amount of air may be seen as it is being swallowed.

Contrast Examination of the Esophagus – Esophagram

Indications

✓ Regurgitation

✓ Dysphagia

✓ Mediastinal masses

✓ Dilated esophagus on survey

Considerations for Contrast Exam of Esophagus

✓ Contrast medium must coat the esophageal mucosa to provide residual contrast that can be seen on the radiographs.

✓ Use a commercially prepared barium paste.

✓ Use iodine contrast media instead of barium if a perforation is suspected. Remember that iodine will not coat, and a small lesion may be missed. If a perforation is not seen with iodine, repeat the procedure with barium.

✓ An esophagram is quick and easy to perform.

✓ No preparation or sedation is required.

✓ Remember to expose survey radiographs prior to using contrast.

Esophagram Technique

1. Barium paste

✓ Give 5-15 ml barium paste orally with a tongue depressor or syringe, or by squeezing the tube into the mouth.

✓ Use a high density paste, not the liquid barium sulfate suspension. Paste is safer if aspirated as it mixes well with fluid and flows around intraluminal structures. Expose lateral and ventrodorsal oblique radiographs immediately after the paste is swallowed.

2. "Barium burger"

✓ Mix liquid barium suspension with canned dog food.

✓ Most dogs will eat the mixture voluntarily.

✓ It evaluates the animal's ability to swallow solid material.

✓ Expose the lateral and ventrodorsal films immediately after the dog eats.

✓ Use the "barium burger" if the esophagram with barium paste is normal.

✓ Use the "barium burger" after the esophagram with barium paste to get additional information.

Normal Esophagram

♥ Fine linear striations are seen from cricopharyngeus to cardia in dogs (Figure 5-1).

✓ Irregularity of mucosal folds at thoracic inlet as normal variation may be seen in dogs.

♥ In cats, transverse striations are in caudal one-third of esophagus–herringbone pattern (Figure 5-2).

💣 If you see a small dilated area, it may represent a bolus being swallowed, so repeat the exposure.

Figure 5-1
Lateral view shows a normal esophagram in a dog.

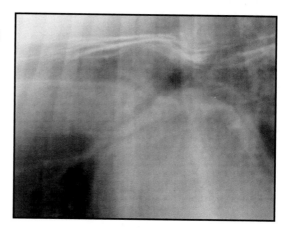

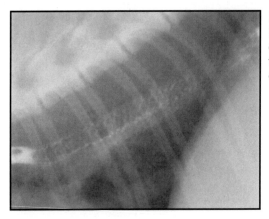

Figure 5-2
Lateral view shows a normal esophagram in a cat. Notice the herringbone pattern in the distal esophagus.

Disorders of the Esophagus

Esophageal Foreign Bodies

✓ Radiopaque foreign bodies can be seen (Figure 5-3). ⊙

✓ Some fluid-opaque foreign bodies are surrounded by air and can be seen (Figure 5-4).

💣✴ If gas is seen in the mediastinum concurrent with an esophageal foreign body, suspect perforation. Some esophageal foreign bodies can penetrate and migrate into the pleural space resulting in pleural effusion (see Figure 5-3D).

Megaesophagus

✓ Idiopathic megaesophagus can be congenital or acquired.

✓ Regurgitation is typical but the owner may confuse regurgitation and vomiting.

Roentgen Signs

✓ The enlarged esophagus is distended with gas or ingesta (Figure 5-5).

✓ The presence of luminal gas may allow the esophageal wall to be seen.

✓ Ventral displacement of the trachea and heart.

♥ Concurrent aspiration pneumonia may be present.

✓ A diverticulum may form in the cranium mediastinum (Figure 5-6). The diverticulum may fill with rotting food, which can be unpleasant if the dog belches!

✔ The use of a barium burger can help diagnose questionable cases of esophageal dysfunction (Figure 5-7). ⊙

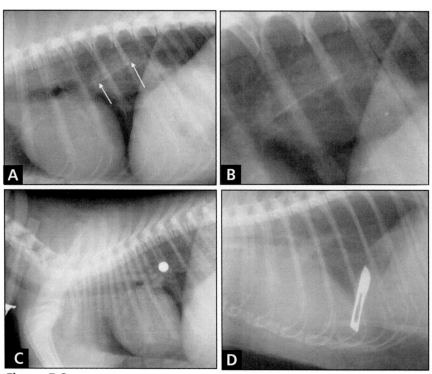

Figure 5-3
Radiopaque esophageal foreign bodies. **A.** Lateral view of a chicken bone (between the white arrows) in the distal esophagus. **B.** Close-up of the chicken bone in Figure 5-3A. **C.** What is this metallic foreign body? **D.** A scalpel blade perforated through the esophagus into the pleural space, creating pleural effusion.

Figure 5-4
Lateral view of the esophagus of a dog shows gristle (arrows) in the esophagus. Air outlining the fluid-opaque gristle allows visualization of this foreign body.

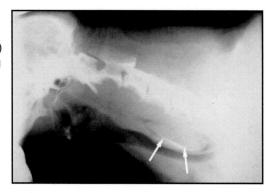

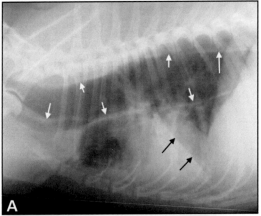

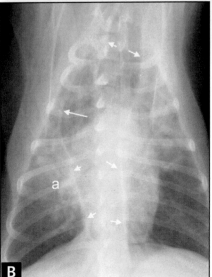

Figure 5-5
A 6-year old Cocker Spaniel with a 2 week history of vomiting and depression. Radiographs show a gas-filled enlarged esophagus; the final diagnosis was myasthenia gravis. Notice alveolar disease in the right middle lung lobe, which is likely associated with aspiration secondary to regurgitation. Black arrows: caudal edge of the right middle lung lobe; white arrows: margins of the gas-filled esophagus; T: trachea (displaced ventrally); a: air bronchogram. **A.** Lateral view. **B.** Ventrodorsal view.

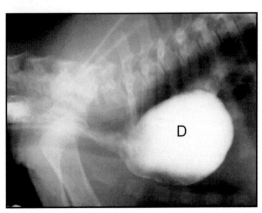

Figure 5-6
Lateral view of the thorax of a dog with megaesophagus shows an associated diverticulum (D).

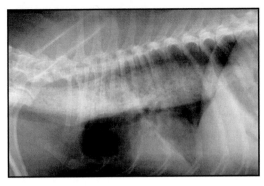

Figure 5-7
Lateral view of the thorax of the dog in Figure 5-5 after the dog ate dog food mixed with barium (barium burger).

Vascular Ring Anomalies

✓ A vascular anomaly can encircle and constrict the esophagus (Figure 5-8). ⊙

✓ The most common anomaly is called the "persistent right aortic arch" (PRAA).

Roentgen Signs

Lateral

> ✓ You may see enlarged gas- or food-filled esophagus.
>
> ✓ Enlargement is cranial or both cranial and caudal to a constriction at the heart base.
>
> ✓ Look for aspiration pneumonia.
>
> ✓ If necessary, confirm the anomaly with an esophagram.

Ventrodorsal

> ✓ Cranial mediastinum may appear widened.
>
> ✓ Enlarged gas or food-filled esophagus may be seen.
>
> ✓ PRAA: the trachea may be pushed to the left by a dense mass (the right aortic arch) in the cranial mediastinum.

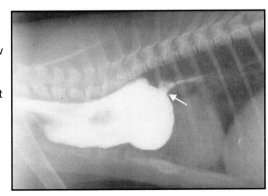

Figure 5-8
Lateral esophagram in a dog shows megaesophagus. Arrow indicates constriction of the esophagus at the heart base secondary to a persistent right aortic arch.

Esophageal Masses

Extramural (Periesophageal)

Roentgen Signs

✓ Displacement of esophagus but normal linear striations on esophagram.

Examples are

- ✓ Lymphadenopathy
- ✓ Granulomas
- ✓ Tumors
- ✓ Enlarged heart

Intramural (within esophageal wall)

Roentgen Signs

✓ Retention of barium paste

✓ Rigid esophageal wall

♥ Filling defect in barium caused by mass

✓ Acquired strictures can result from severe chronic esophagitis.

Examples are

- ✓ Neoplasia
- ✓ Fibrosis

✓ Parasitic granuloma (Figure 5-9). ⊙ *Spirocerca lupi* is a parasite whose larvae migrate between the esophagus and aorta. Granuloma causes opacity in the caudo-dorsal thorax. Spondylosis may be seen along the caudal thoracic vertebrae.

✓ Chronic esophagitis. May be a reaction to a foreign body. Reflux esophagitis is a reaction to gastric acids.

Intraluminal

Roentgen Signs

✓ Retention of barium paste

✓ Barium flows around intraluminal mass

♥ Filling defect

Examples are

- ✓ Foreign bodies
- ✓ Tumors

✓ Broncho-esophageal fistulas can occur secondary to esophageal foreign bodies. A classic sign is coughing after drinking liquid.

May be a fluid radiopacity in lung

Esophagram shows contrast flowing from the esophageal lumen to the lung opacity.

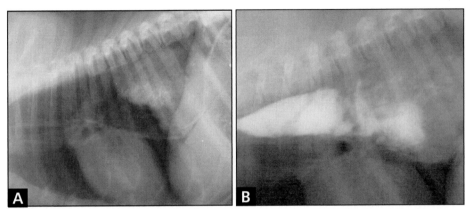

Figure 5-9
Radiographs of a dog with an intramural esophageal mass caused by the parasite *Spirocerca lupi*. **A.** Lateral view shows a mass in the caudodorsal thorax. **B.** Esophagram shows that the mass is an intramural esophageal mass.

Radiography of the Stomach and Small Intestine

Survey Radiographs

✓ Remember to expose survey radiographs prior to contrast radiograph.

✓ Gas is normally seen in the gastrointestinal tract.

✓ The diameter of the small intestine should not exceed:

Dogs – 2x the diameter of a rib or the height of the central part of a vertebra.

Cats – 2x the height of the central part of L4 or 12 mm.

✓ If a radiopaque foreign body is seen, check for evidence of perforation or obstruction.

Contrast Examination of the Stomach and Small Intestine – Indications

✓ Vomiting

✓ Small bowel diarrhea

✓ Organ displacement

✓ Abdominal masses

Upper Gastrointestinal Series

✓ Contrast examination of stomach and small intestine with positive contrast media.

✓ Also called a "barium series" because the usual contrast medium is barium.

Technique

✓ Perform a thorough preparation of the gastrointestinal tract

24-hour fast

Laxatives

Enemas should be given at least 1-2 hours before the study to allow for expulsion of gas and fluid that is typically in the colon immediately after an enema.

Withhold drinking water 1-2 hours before to avoid a fluid-filled stomach.

💣※ Expose survey radiographs immediately before contrast radiography.

To determine if ingesta or other extraneous materials in or on the patient may interfere with the contrast study (Figure 5-10)

Might yield diagnostic information not present on previous survey films that could obviate the need for the contrast study.

Do not proceed if not adequately prepared

✓ Administer barium suspension orally or by stomach tube.

Contrast Medium: Liquid barium suspensions

✓ United States Pharmacopoeia (U.S.P.) barium mixed with water has been used but the U.S.P. barium precipitates and flocculates.

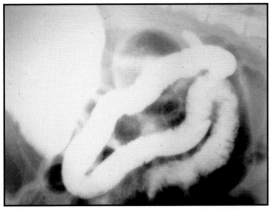

Figure 5-10
Lateral view of the abdomen of a dog that ingested lead paint. The radiopaque paint would not be apparent if survey radiography was not performed.

✓ Commercially prepared suspensions 30% weight per volume (w/v) stay in suspension.

☙ Commercially-prepared micro-fine barium suspension is contrast medium of choice for upper GI series.

Barium Dose
♥ 6 cc/lb = 1 oz/5 lb. A full dose is necessary to distend the stomach and stimulate gastric emptying.

Technique
♥ Standard abdominal technique PLUS 6-8 kVp

Film Sequence in Dogs
✓ Make frequent films during first hour. Observe stomach, gastric emptying, and proximal small intestine.

✓ A lesion in the small intestine will slow transit. The interval between films should be increased to compensate for the slower transit time. Tailor the sequence to the individual!

✓ Always continue series until the stomach empties and barium reaches the colon unless a firm diagnosis is made before the barium arrives there.

Typical Sequence

Immediate	1 hour		
15 minutes	2 hours		
30 minutes	4 hours		

**always two projections (ventro-dorsal, lateral) at each time

At 18 to 24 hours, a final radiograph the "morning after" is frequently useful, particularly if the stomach has not emptied.

Keys to Good Upper GI Series

✔ Proper preparation

✔ Use liquid barium suspension if possible

✔ Use adequate dose

✔ Take enough films

Complications

1. Inhalation of barium

✔ Barium is inert and nonirritating

✔ Barium in trachea or main stem bronchi will be removed by ciliary action and coughing within a few hours with no permanent problem.

✔ Barium in alveoli: Small amount (Figure 5-11) will wall off and remain in lung and will be visible years later. Animal will recover and will probably have no clinical signs.

✔ Barium in alveoli: Large amount (entire lobe or lung): Grave prognosis

2. Intractable patient

♥ Excited or frightened patient usually has decreased GI motility

✔ Sympathetic stimulation (fight or flight). Take time to handle and position animal gently.

✔ It's preferable not to use any chemical restraint.

✔ If drugs are necessary, the preferred drugs include a small dose of acepromazine in dogs, or a small dose of ketamine/diazepam in cats because they have a minimal effect on GI motility .

3. Current therapy

✔ Antiemetic and antidiarrheal drugs markedly alter GI motility.

✔ Withdraw such medication 48-72 hours before the GI series, if possible.

Normal Upper GI Series

Stomach

✔ Fully distended stomach

Rugal folds in fundus may be distinctive (Figure 5-12)

Contractions occur normally in the stomach

Figure 5-11
Lateral radiograph taken after accidental inhalation of barium shows alveolarization of barium.

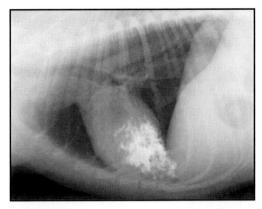

Figure 5-12
Dorsoventral view of the stomach of a dog with barium shows prominent rugal folds (white arrows) and a normal gastric contraction (black arrow).

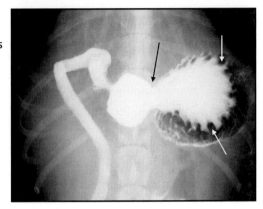

✓ Differences occur because of positioning:

☞ Barium suspension is liquid and liquid runs downhill

✓ Be able to recognize which position is shown

✓ Expose films using all four projections especially when gastric disease is suspected.

Left Lateral Recumbent Position

   ✓ Contrast fills and distends fundus and body (Figure 5-13)

   ✓ Gas rises to the pyloric antrum

Right Lateral Recumbent Position

   ✓ Contrast fills and distends pyloric antrum and part of body (Figure 5-14)

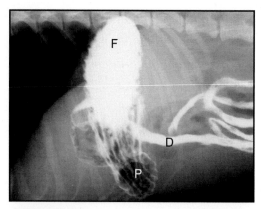

Figure 5-13
Normal upper gastrointestinal series of a dog in left lateral recumbency shows barium in the fundus (F) and body, and gas in the pylorus antrum (P). D: duodenum.

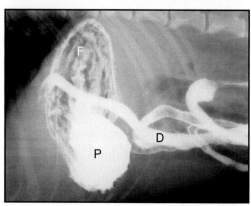

Figure 5-14
Normal upper gastrointestinal series of a dog in right lateral recumbency shows barium in the pyloric antrum (P) and part of the body, and gas in the fundus (F). D: duodenum.

✔ The most helpful way to differentiate the ventrodorsal and dorsoventral views is to look at the gastric body.

Dorsal Recumbency–Ventrodorsal View

✔ Gas is mainly in the body.

✔ Barium is in the fundus and pylorus (Figure 5-15).

✔ Fundus may continue to trap gas and may contain both barium and gas.

Ventral Recumbency–Dorsoventral View

✔ Barium seen mainly in gastric body and pylorus (Figure 5-16)

✔ Gas is mainly in the fundus (some barium will be in the ventral portion).

Small Intestine

♥ Barium appears as a continuous column or ribbon

✓ Normal small intestine shows "feathered" edge (intestinal villi)

✓ Lymphoid follicles (Peyer's patches) are normal and should not be interpreted as ulcers (Figure 5-17). ⊙

✓ Segmental contractions should be present

Figure 5-15
Normal upper gastrointestinal series of dog in dorsal recumbency (ventrodorsal view) shows gas mainly in the body (B) and barium in the pylorus (P). Notice that the fundus (F) continues to trap gas even in this position so that both barium and gas are seen in the fundus. D:duodenum.

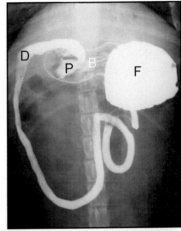

Figure 5-16
Normal upper gastrointestinal series of a dog in ventral recumbency (dorsoventral view) shows barium in the body (B), pylorus and the ventral portion of the fundus, and gas in the dorsal portion of the fundus (F). D:duodenum; P:pyloric antrum.

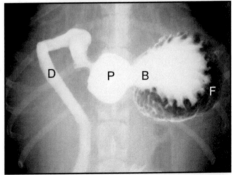

Figure 5-17
Normal upper gastrointestinal series of a dog shows Peyer's patches (arrows) in the descending duodenum (D). A:ascending duodenum.

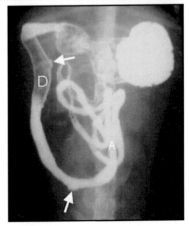

Differences in Cats

✓ Remember the stomach is J-shaped (Figure 5-18).

✓ Normal hypersegmentation in the duodenum give the duodenum a "string of pearls" appearance.

✓ Barium will reach the colon within 30-60 minutes.

✓ By 90 minutes, most of the barium will be in the colon (Figure 5-19).

✓ The faster transit time necessitates more frequent exposures over a shorter period of time than needed for dogs.

✓ The cecum is nonsacculated and comma-shaped.

Principles of Interpretation

✓ Remember that the GI tract is constantly in motion.

✓ We see only "stop-action pictures."

☛ True anatomic abnormalities persist on sequential radiographs.

✓ If you suspect a mucosal lesion, look for repeatability .

♥ Most upper GI series do not yield a specific diagnosis.

✓ Chronic vomiting and diarrhea often has metabolic or functional etiology without anatomic disease.

✓ Some principles answer important questions:

> Is anatomic disease present?
>
> Is there mucosal involvement?
>
> Is there infiltrative disease?
>
> Is there intraluminal or extraluminal disease?
>
> Is a lesion focal or diffuse?
>
> Where is the lesion located?
>
> Is the lesion obstructive or nonobstructive?

✓ An intestinal biopsy is often required for specific or etiologic diagnosis.

✓ Occasionally a specific diagnosis is made.

✓ Occasionally a cure is realized because of the therapeutic value of barium.

Other Contrast Procedures

Upper GI Series with Iodine

✓ Use organic iodine contrast if a perforation is suspected.

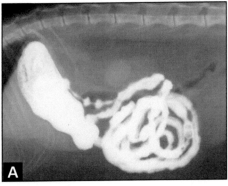

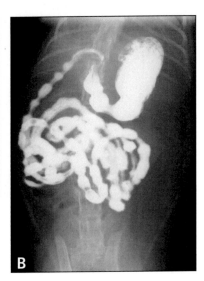

Figure 5-18
Normal upper gastrointestinal series of a cat 15 minutes after administering barium. Notice the J-shaped stomach in the dorsoventral view and the "string of pearls" effect in both views. **A.** Lateral view. **B.** Dorsoventral view.

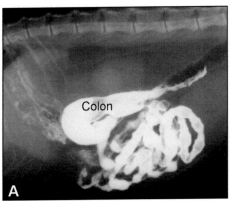

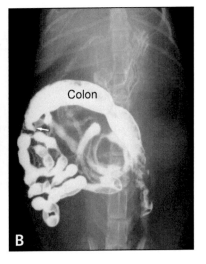

Figure 5-19
Normal upper gastrointestinal series of a cat 90 minutes after administrating barium. Barium has already reached the colon. Arrow: cecum. **A.** Lateral view. **B.** Dorsoventral view.

✓ The transit is fast, so take radiographs more frequently (Figure 5-20).

✓ Iodine does not coat as well as barium.

✓ Hypertonicity causes dilution of the iodine so the study will appear blurred.

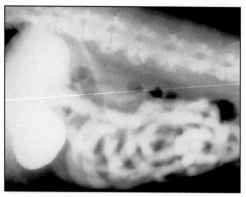

Figure 5-20
Normal upper gastrointestinal series of a dog using a water-soluble iodine contrast agent instead of barium.

Pneumogastrogram

✓ This is a negative contrast study of the stomach.

✓ This procedure is quick and easy.

✓ Radiograph the abdomen after passing a stomach tube and inflating the stomach to slight-to-moderate tympany.

✓ A quick screen for radiolucent gastric foreign body or to determine the stomach's position.

Double Contrast Gastrogram

✓ An empty stomach is required; fasting is necessary.

✓ Administer 10-20 ml liquid barium suspension.

✓ Inflate the stomach with air.

✓ Make multiple radiographic projections.

✓ This method is excellent to evaluate gastric mucosa, gastric neoplasia, and ulceration.

✓ This method is also excellent for coating of gastric foreign bodies.

Disorders of the Stomach

Gastric Foreign Body

✓ Some gastric foreign bodies are radiopaque and identifiable with a little imagination (Figure 5-21).

✓ If a gastric foreign body is suspected but not seen on survey radiographs, administer a small amount of barium (10-20 ml) in an attempt to coat the object

✓Take all four views (ventrodorsal, dorsoventral, right lateral, left lateral)

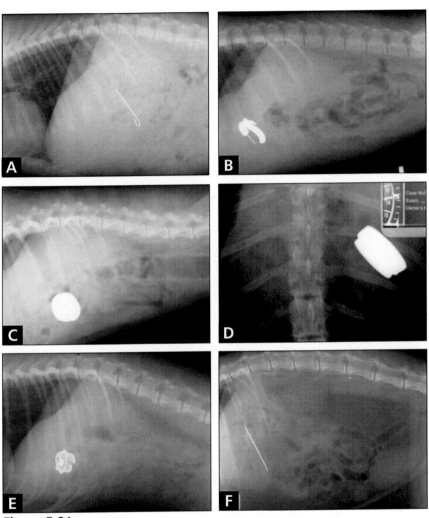

Figure 5-21
A. Did you recognize the esophageal foreign body in Figure 5-3C? Hint: he swallowed it, hook, line, and sinker! **B.** Someone must be missing an earring. **C.** This foreign body is difficult to recognize in one image. **D.** In the ventrodorsal view, the foreign body in Figure 5-21C is actually several coins. **E.** "Jingle bells, jingle bells, jingle all the way..." **F.** "A stitch in time..."

✔ If results are negative, administer a full dose of barium and look for a filling defect (Figure 5-22A). If results are still negative, proceed to a full GI series.

☕ "Morning after" film may show retention of barium (Figure 5-22B). ⊙

✔ Gas in the stomach, either naturally occurring or that appears after a pneumogastrogram is performed, can outline a foreign body (Figure 5-23). ⊙

Gastric Torsion/Dilatation

Roentgen Signs

✔ The stomach is distended in both conditions.

✔ Expose both lateral views for comparison.

✔ The right lateral recumbent view is most helpful:

♥ In right lateral recumbency, a normally positioned pyloric antrum will be located ventrally on the right side. It will be fluid-filled even when the stomach is dilated (Figure 5-24). ⊙

☕ Most commonly in torsion (Figure 5-25):

> The pylorus moves from ventral right, travels along the ventral abdomen to the left (clockwise rotation when the animal is viewed from behind). In the right lateral recumbent view, the pylorus will be gas filled and located dorsally, cranial to the fundus,

💣 **BUT** direction and degree of torsion is variable.

> For example, the stomach may rotate clockwise in a full circle. The pylorus will be positioned normally.

> Rarely, the pylorus may travel dorsally along the right side to become located dorsally on the right side. (In the LEFT lateral recumbent view, the pylorus will be gas-filled and located dorsally, cranial to the fundus.)

Pyloric Outflow Obstruction

Causative Conditions

Pyloric stenosis (Figure 5-26)

Pylorospasm

Inflammation

Hypertrophy

Scar Tissue

Neoplasia (Figure 5-27)

Foreign Body

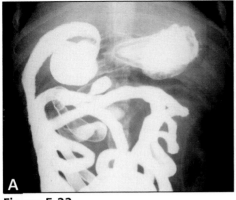

Figure 5-22
A. Upper GI series of a 5-year old dog 3 hours after barium administration. The filling defect was caused by a dog leash in the stomach. **B.** After 20 hours, barium can be seen in the colon and cecum but is still retained in the stomach.

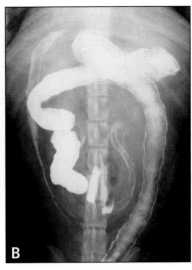

Figure 5-23
Left lateral recumbent view shows gastrointestinal gas outlining a piece of beach towel in the stomach (white arrows) and duodenum (black arrows) of an Irish Wolfhound with dietary indiscretion.

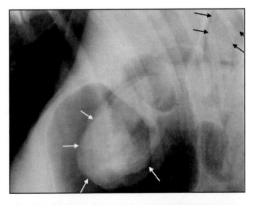

Figure 5-24
Right lateral recumbent view of the abdomen of a Doberman Pinscher with gastric dilatation without torsion. The pylorus is ventral, fluid-filled, and not clearly visible in this radiograph.

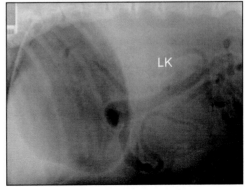

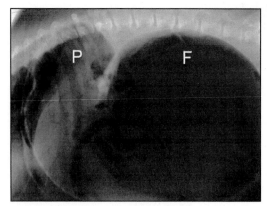

Figure 5-25
Right lateral recumbent view of the abdomen of a Chow Chow with gastric torsion. (P) The pylorus is located dorsally, cranial to the fundus (F).

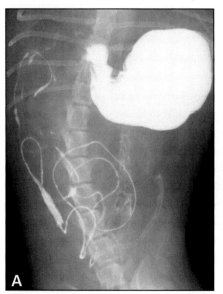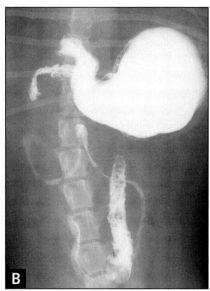

Figure 5-26
Pyloric outflow obstruction in a 5-year old Pekingese with hypertrophied pyloric mucosal folds. **A.** Ventrodorsal view 2 hours after barium administration. Notice that most of the barium is retained in the stomach, and only a thin ribbon of contrast is seen in the proximal small intestine. **B.** Ventrodorsal view at 5 hours. Although some barium reached the colon, contrast remains in the stomach.

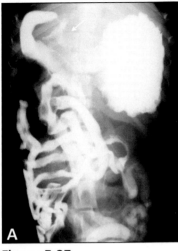 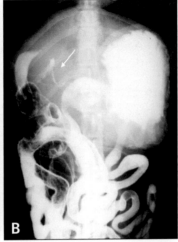

Figure 5-27
Ventrodorsal views of the stomach of a dog with chronic weight loss caused by gastric adenocarcinoma and consequent pyloric outflow obstruction. Notice the rigidity and lack of change in the contrast column in the area of the mass (arrow) **A.** 3.5 hours after barium administration. **B.** 6 hours after barium administration. **C.** Radiograph of another dog with gastric adenocarci-

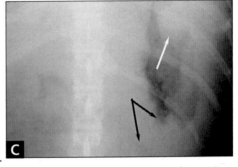

noma showing gas outlining the irregular mass (white arrow). Ultrasonography confirmed increased wall thickness caused by the neoplasm (black arrows).

Roentgen Signs in Survey Films

♥ The stomach is typically distended with fluid.

✓ Might see opacity at the pylorus with foreign body or neoplasia.

✓ Note that air can be used to outline a foreign body or other lesion.

Roentgen Signs in Upper GI Series

✓ Delayed gastric emptying

✓ Pyloric neoplasia may show as a persistent asymmetric filling defect at the pylorus.

✓ Cloth foreign body:

+/- filling defect in the barium contrast

Barium is retained by the material even after most of the contrast has reached the colon.

Take films the next day with slow gastric emptying (see Figure 5-22)

Gastric Neoplasia

The most common gastric neoplasms are adenocarcinoma in dogs and lymphosarcoma in cats. Their appearance varies with size, shape, and location.

Roentgen Signs in Survey Films

✓ The normal gastric gas may outline a mass.

✓ The normal gas bubble in the fundus may be distorted or malpositioned (see Figure 5-27C).

✓ Masses at the pylorus may result in pyloric outflow obstruction (see Figure 5-27).

✓ A large mass may be difficult to distinguish from a full stomach or liver mass.

Roentgen Signs in Upper GI Series

✓ Filling defect is seen if the mass is sufficiently large.

♥ Rigidity of the gastric wall or irregularity of the barium contrast.

✓ Delayed gastric emptying if the mass is at the pylorus causing outflow obstruction.

✓ Wall thickening.

Gastroesophageal Intussusception

✓ The stomach is pushed into the lumen of the esophagus.

✓ The intussusception can cause obstruction resulting in dilation of the stomach.

💣 This may present as a medical emergency.

✓ Differential diagnosis is hiatal hernia (see page 32)

Roentgen Signs in Survey Films

✓ Lateral view: fluid opacity is seen in the caudo-dorsal thorax (Figure 5-28)

✓ Ventro-dorsal view: fluid opacity is seen centrally cranial to the diaphragm

✓ Air might be in the fluid opacity

Roentgen Signs in Upper GI Series

✓ Barium outlines the displaced rugal folds in the caudal esophagus.

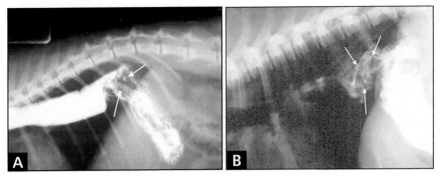

Figure 5-28
Lateral views. **A.** A young cat with gastroesophageal intussusception. **B.** A young Boston Terrier with gastroesophageal intussusception presented for regurgitation. In the case of the cat, the intussusception was intermittent and could be demonstrated by elevating the hindquarters. Arrows indicate rugal folds in the esophagus.

Disorders of the Small Intestine

Ileus

✓ Motility of the bowel is decreased or completely stopped.

✓ The ileus can be functional or mechanical.

✓ The "sentinel" loop is a dilated loop that signals an area of disease (e.g., gas in the duodenum may indicate peritonitis secondary to pancreatitis).

Roentgen Signs in Survey Films

✓ Intestinal walls become rigid and parallel.

✓ Gas- or fluid-filled loop(s) of small intestine exceed the diameter of a rib by 3 to 4 times.

✓ Dilation can be localized or generalized, and either mild to severe.

✓ Severe dilation could indicate obstruction (e.g., foreign body, volvulus).

✓ Severe generalized dilation could be functional or could be caused by a distal obstruction or volvulus around the mesenteric root.

✓ Generalized or mild dilation could be caused by enteritis or aerophagia. Consider clinical signs.

Mechanical Obstruction

✓ History of painful abdomen

Roentgen Signs in Survey Films

☗ Dilation of small intestine is proximal to obstruction (Figure 5-29). ⊙ The obstruction is seen as gas or, less commonly, fluid-filled loops of small intestine.

✓ "Stacked" (multiple parallel loops) loops of small intestine (Figure 5-29)

✓ The intestine is compressed at the turns ("hairpin" turns).

✓ May see cause of obstruction (e.g., mass, foreign body)

✓ The cause is not always seen.

Roentgen Signs in Upper GI Series

♥ Barium fills the dilated segment of bowel proximal to obstruction (Figure 5-30).

✓ The cause of the obstruction may be seen as a filling defect in the contrast column.

♥ Occasionally a foreign body takes up the barium and can be better seen the next day (Figure 5-30).

Foreign Body

Roentgen Signs in Survey Films

✓ Metallic or mineral foreign bodies will be visible.

💣 If sharp metal foreign bodies are seen, check for evidence of perforation (Figures 5-31 and 5-32).

✓ Some fluid opaque foreign bodies will have a typical shape or pattern especially when outlined by air (Figure 5-33).

✓ String foreign bodies are common in cats.

   ♥ Typically, you will see accordion-like bowel or plicated, gathered loops of bowel (Figure 5-34). ⊙

   ✓ Don't confuse the normal "string of pearls" appearance of the feline duodenum with a string foreign body.

   ✓ Remember to check under cat's tongue for the string!

   ✓ There may be signs of obstruction as noted above.

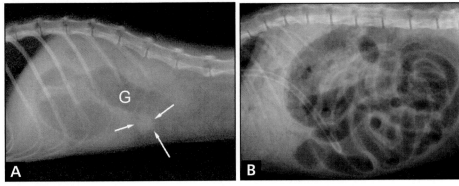

Figure 5-29
A. Lateral view of the abdomen of a cat with an intestinal foreign body in the proximal small intestine. A dilated gas-filled loop of small intestine (G) is seen proximal to the foreign body (arrows). **B.** Lateral view of a different cat with a distal foreign body causing generalized severe distension of the small intestine with gas. Multiple parallel loops of gas-filled bowel are apparent. A nasogastric tube was placed into the stomach to relieve distension and stabilize the patient prior to surgery.

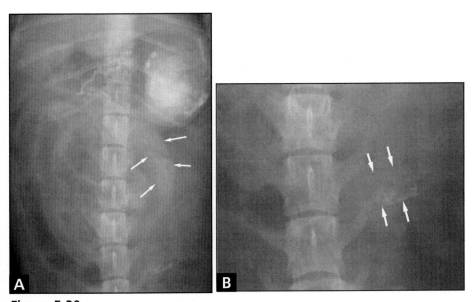

Figure 5-30
Upper GI series in a 6 month old Dachshund with a jejunal foreign body. **A.** Ventro-dorsal view shows barium in a dilated loop of small intestine (arrows) proximal to the obstruction. **B.** The next day, the foreign body (arrows) is outlined by barium.

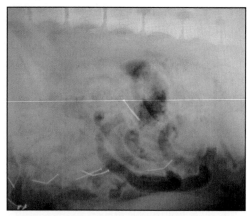

Figure 5-31
Lateral view of the abdomen of a dog who feasted on dog biscuits that were pinned to a Christmas wreath. There are multiple intestinal foreign bodies (pins and more pins). Notice that serosal detail is good; no extraluminal gas is apparent. The pins passed uneventfully.

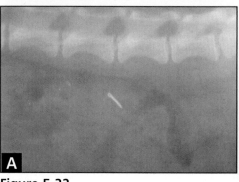

Figure 5-32
Radiographs of the abdomen of dog showing a needle (note the hole at the end) in the small intestine. **A.** In the lateral view, the needle appears fairly small because it's seen end-on. **B.** The ventrodorsal view reveals the needle's, actual length. Surgery revealed that the needle was protruding through the intestinal wall at the caudal duodenal flexure.

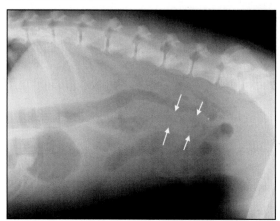

Figure 5-33
Corncob foreign bodies (arrows) typically are somewhat rectangular with a pitted surface. A lucent core may be visualized

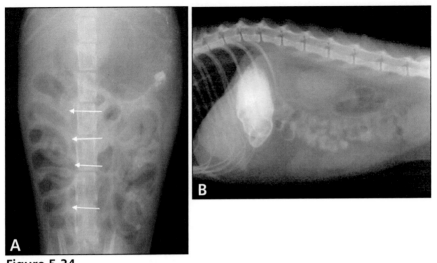

Figure 5-34
String foreign body in two cats. **A.** Gas in this cat's duodenum shows the typical accordion-like pattern of string foreign body in the intestine. Arrows indicate the mesenteric border along which the intestine is gathered. **B.** Contrast radiography with iodine (in case of perforation) clearly demonstrates the typical pattern in this cat.

Roentgen Signs in Upper GI Series

✓ A foreign body frequently shows as a filling defect in barium contrast (Figure 5-35).

✓ An intestinal cloth foreign body has an appearance similar to a gastric cloth foreign body.

✓ If contrast is needed to confirm string foreign bodies, iodine contrast should be used because of the danger of perforation (see Figure 5-34B).

Intussusception

✓ Intussusception of the small intestine commonly results in obstruction.

✓ The telescoped loop of bowel is the intussusceptum; the receiving loop is the intussuscipiens.

✓ There may be a palpable sausage-like mass.

Roentgen Signs in Survey Films

✓ Gas- or fluid-filled distended loops of bowel indicate obstruction.

✓ Fluid opacity may be present at the site of the intussusception.

✓ Gas may outline the intussusceptum.

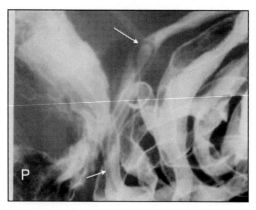

Figure 5-35
Round worm shows up as filling defect (arrows) in the barium contrast column in this dog. P:pylorus.

Roentgen Signs in Upper GI Series

✓ May be delayed transit associated with ileus

♥ Intussusceptum shows as a filling defect within the contrast column.

Inflammatory Diseases Without Ulceration

Roentgen Signs in Survey Films

May appear normal, with variable amounts of gas.

Roentgen Signs in Upper GI Series

✓ Transit time may be faster

✓ Mild irregularity of the mucosal surface may be seen.

✓ Barium may layer on the bowel wall if a lot of mucus is present (snake skin appearance).

✓ The lumen width may be decreased.

Ulcers

✓ Ulcers may be associated with neoplasms, granulomatous disease, parasites, uremia, or administration of nonsteroidal anti-inflammatory drugs.

Roentgen Signs in Survey Films

✓ May not be able to appreciate lesion in survey radiography especially if the animal is emaciated.

Roentgen Signs in Upper GI Series

✓ A pocket or crater can be seen in the intestinal wall.

✔ Asymmetry, undermining of mucosa, and rigidity help differentiate true ulcers from Peyer's patches.

Infiltrative Disease
(Figures 5-36, 5-37, and 5-38)

Neoplasia, Mycosis, Plasmacytic-lymphocytic Enteritis
✔ A biopsy is necessary for differentiation of these diseases.

✔ The most common neoplasms are adenocarcinoma and lymphosarcoma.

✔ Neoplasms can also present as localized masses (Figure 5-38); see also page 51.

Roentgen Signs on Survey Films
✔ Mast cell tumors may be associated with ulceration of the small intestine.

✔ Adenocarcinomas typically cause concentric wall thickening, resulting in decreased size of the lumen and partial or complete obstruction.

✔ Lymphosarcoma in cats causes wall thickening that may or may not be concentric.

✔ Lymphosarcoma in dogs is more likely to cause a focal patchy thickening that is not concentric.

♥ Signs of infiltrative disease include

Dilated bowel proximal to the affected area

"Applecore" lesions are seen in which the lumen is narrow and the mucosa is irregular

Fixed spicules on the borders of the contrast column

A mass-like effect is seen with displacement of other parts of the gastrointestinal tract

The lumens of affected portions of the intestine narrow

Pneumatosis Intestinalis
✔ Refers to gas in the submucosa of the intestine (Figure 5-39)

✔ A similar condition in the colon is termed pneumatosis coli.

✔ It may resolve spontaneously.

Roentgen Signs
♥ Lucency is seen within the intestinal wall.

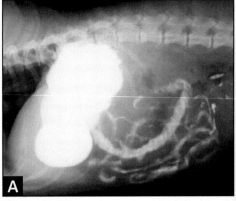

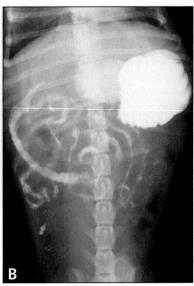

Figure 5-36
Upper GI series in a dog with plasmacytic-lymphocytic enteritis, a diffuse infiltrative disease. Notice irregularity and narrowing of affected areas of the small intestine. **A.** Lateral view at 15 minutes. **B.** Ventrodorsal view at 15 minutes.

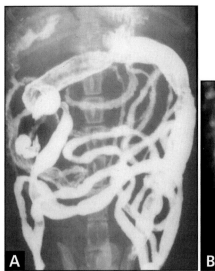

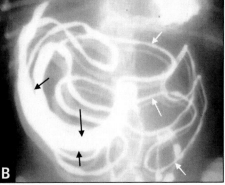

Figure 5-37
A. Ventrodorsal view of an upper GI series of a dog with histoplasmosis. Affected areas are narrowed and irregular (arrows). **B.** Multiple areas are narrowed (white arrows) secondary to intestinal adenocarcinoma in this 13-year old Cairn Terrier 30 minutes after oral administration of contrast medium. Other areas appear dilated (black arrows).

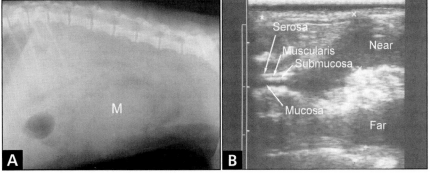

Figure 5-38
Intestinal mass in a dog. **A.** Lateral view. **B.** Sonogram of an intestinal mass in a dog. Normal wall layers are seen in the adjacent normal small intestine. In the area of the mass, wall layers can not be identified in the near and far wall.

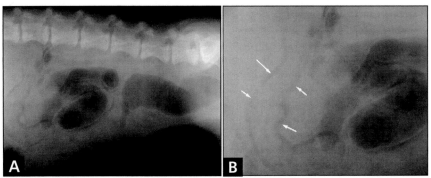

Figure 5-39
Pneumatosis intestinalis in a dog. **A.** Lateral radiograph. **B.** Close-up lateral radiograph with arrows indicating gas in the intestinal wall.

Radiography of the Large Intestine

Survey Radiographs

✓ A normal colon has a "shepherd's crook" shape.

✓ The cecum in the dog is a pig's tail shape.

✓ The cecum in the cat is a comma shape.

Contrast Radiography of the Large Intestine

✔ Pneumocolography is the procedure of choice.

✔ A barium enema is a complex procedure that requires anesthesia. Endoscopy has largely replaced use of the barium enema.

Pneumocolography

Indications

✔ Suspected ileocolic intussusception or cecal inversion

✔ Need to differentiate between the large versus small intestine

✔ May aid in identification of strictures or masses

✔ Mucosal lesions are better examined with a barium enema, colonoscopy, or ultrasound.

Technique

♥ Quick and easy procedure

Fill a 30-60 ml syringe with air

Place the syringe tip in the anus and press the front of syringe barrel against the anus to seal.

Slowly instill air

Repeat to fill colon 5-10 ml/lb (30 ml for a small dog; up to 200-300 ml for a large dog).

✔ Make ventro-dorsal and lateral radiographs, obliques if necessary.

Normal Appearance

Gas smoothly fills the ascending colon, transverse colon, and descending colon (Figure 5-40).

Barium Enema

✔ Oral barium usually does not allow adequate evaluation of the colon.

Indications

Large bowel diarrhea

Tenesmus

Rectal bleeding

Indeterminate signs of colon disease on survey radiographs are: decreased lumen diameter; shortening of the colon; strictures; and thickened wall.

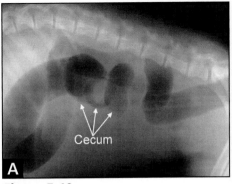

Figure 5-40
Contrast radiography in the large bowel.
A. Normal lateral pneumocologram. **B.**
Normal ventrodorsal pneumocologram.

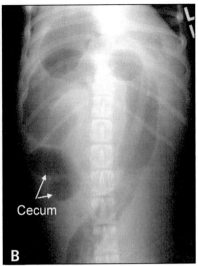

Technique

Preparation

✓ Thorough preparation of the colon is essential; it must be squeaky clean.

> Withhold food for at least 24 hours
>
> Give laxatives and enemas the evening before the exam
>
> 1-2 hours before exam, give a warm water enema until the fluid is clear
>
> Do not give an enema immediately before the exam because it introduces gas and fluid artifact

✓ General anesthesia is required: canine and feline patients will not cooperate, even under sedation.

✓ Obtain survey radiographs immediately before contrast administration (scout films). If the colon is not fully prepared, do not proceed.

Contrast

✓ Contrast medium is a liquid barium suspension (30% w/v) diluted 1:1 with warm water.

✓ Administer 5-15 ml/lb via rectal catheter with inflatable cuff. Use bardex catheter or disposable BE (barium enema) catheter with cuff locked snugly in pelvic canal.

✓ Administer barium by gravity flow; barium is in an enema bag suspended from an IV stand.

✓ Give barium until the colon is mildly distended.

✓ If the colon is severely affected, administer 5 cc/lb, radiograph, repeat until 10-15 ml/lb has been given or colon is full to avoid perforation.

✓ In young or debilitated animals where you cannot use a cuff or anesthesia, a syringe can be used to put barium into the colon.

Filming Sequences

✓ Expose a single ventrodorsal radiograph to evaluate the degree of filling.

✓ Barium should not extend into the small intestine. The small intestine fills rapidly and obscures the colon.

✓ If the colon is not filled to cecum, then administer additional barium.

✓ Expose lateral, ventrodorsal, and dorsoventral oblique radiographs of the abdomen. Multiple projections show various profiles of colon wall.

Double Contrast Barium Enema

✓ This procedure is optional.

✓ Remove as much barium as possible from the colon by gravity flow and gentle palpation.

✓ Inflate the colon with air using the rectal catheter.

✓ Radiographs show excellent mucosal detail with barium coating.

Complications

✓ Overinflation of catheter cuff may cause the colon or rectum to tear, especially if the tissue is diseased. Inflate the catheter cuff carefully.

✓ If you suspect a rupture, tear, or perforation of the rectum or colon, do not administer barium sulfate.

💣 Intestinal contents in the peritoneal cavity is a life-threatening situation!

💣 Intestinal contents and barium in the peritoneal cavity causes an even more severe reaction. Immediate surgery is required.

Normal Appearance

✓ The dog's colon is simple, nonsacculated, and has a smooth mucosal lining (see Figure 2-6).

✓ Typically the overall shape is a simple "shepherd's crook."

✓ Additional flexures or folds are present in many normal dogs.

✓ A reflex segmental contraction may be present just cranial to the catheter tip and cuff.

✓ An evaluation of the terminal colon and rectum is impossible with the catheter in place.

✓ If rectal disease is suspected, the catheter should be removed to allow barium to flow into the terminal large intestine.

Disorders of the Large Intestine

Obstipation

Causes

Pelvic fractures

Stricture

Neuromuscular disease

Roentgen Signs

✓ The colon is distended with inspissated fecal material that has increased opacity (Figure 5-41).

Ileocolic Intussusception

✓ Frequently there will be a history of vomiting and weight loss which may have occurred over several weeks.

✓ Sometimes a sausage-like mass can be palpated

✓ The small intestine may be dilated and gas-filled proximal to the obstruction.

Roentgen Signs on Survey Films

✓ Abdomen may be fluid opaque because of emaciation and/or inflammation.

✔ A mass effect may be apparent.

✔ Occasionally, intraluminal colonic gas outlines the intussus-ceptum (telescoped segment of ileum).

Roentgen Signs on Barium Enema

♥ Filling defect in barium contrast column represents the intus-susceptum (Figure 5-42). ⊙

Roentgen Signs on Pneumocolography

♥ Intussusceptum will be seen as a fluid opacity surrounded by air (Figure 5-43).

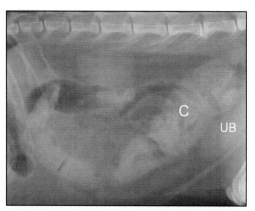

Figure 5-41
Lateral radiograph of the abdomen of a Manx cat with obstipation. C:colon; UB:urinary bladder.

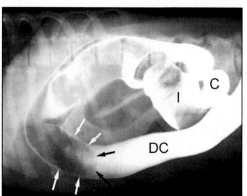

Figure 5-42
Lateral barium enema in a dog with an ileocolic intussusception. The intussusceptum shows as a filling defect (arrows) in the barium in the colon. Note concentric ring appearance where ileum enters cecum. DC:descending colon; I:ileum; C:cecum.

Figure 5-43

Pneumocologram in a 5-month old Boxer with a 2-week history of vomiting, some diarrhea, and weight loss. **A.** Lateral view shows a dilated segment of bowel (arrows) which may be part of either the small or large intestine. **B.** Lateral pneumocologram. Air was injected into the colon using a syringe placed against the anus. Air outlines the distal ileum protruding distally into the colon (ileocolic intussusception). The cecum is a gas-filled structure in the shape of a pig's tail. AC:ascending colon; DC:descending colon. **C.** Ventrodorsal pneumocologram.

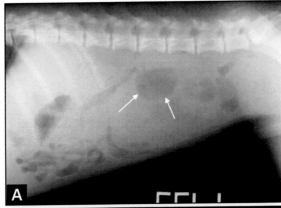

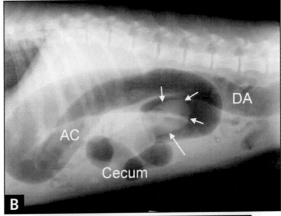

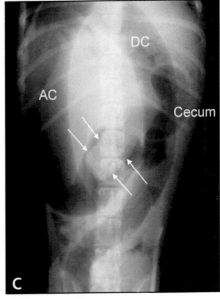

Cecal Inversion

✓ Cecum prolapses into the colon (cecocolic intussusception)

✓ Much less common than ileocolic intussusception

Roentgen Signs

✓ Appearance is similar to that of ileocolic intussusception

✓ Gas-filled cecum will not be visible (Figure 5-44)

✓ Cecal intussusceptum is smaller than an ileal intussusceptum ("thumb-like")

✓ Use pneumocolography and barium enema, just as for ileocolic intussusception

Infiltrative Diseases

History of large bowel diarrhea

Poor prognosis

Examples are

Ulcerative colitis

Granulomatous colitis

Colon or rectal neoplasia

Roentgen Signs on Survey Films

Normal on survey films

Roentgen Signs on Barium Enema

Lumen diameter is decreased

The colon is shortened (Figure 5-45).

Strictures, fistulae

Thickened wall

Mucosal Diseases (Colitis)

✓ History of large bowel diarrhea

✓ Favorable to guarded prognosis depending on severity

Roentgen Signs on Survey Films

Normal on survey films

Roentgen Signs on Barium Enema

✓Mucosal Spicules

Additional signs depending on whether disease is mucosal or transmural

Mucosal	versus	Transmural Disease
1. Serration and spiculation of mucosal pattern		Decreased lumen diameter
2. No shortening		Shortening of colon
3. No strictures, fistulae		Strictures, fistulae, thickened wall
4. Inflammatory		Chronic granulomatous inflammation, neoplasia, fibrosis
5. Favorable/guarded prognosis		Poor prognosis

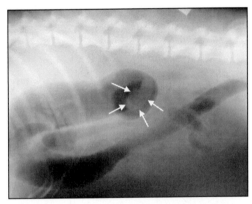

Figure 5-44
Pneumocologram in a dog with cecal inversion. Note the absence of a gas-filled cecum. Arrows indicate the fluid-opaque cecum within the gas-filled colon.

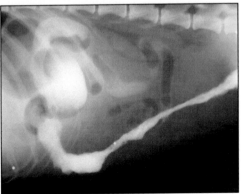

Figure 5-45
Barium enema in a dog with transmural fungal colitis. The contrast column is irregular and thinned. The colonic serosa is not clearly seen.

Non-Ionic Iodinated Contrast Media for Gastrointestinal Studies

Iohexol and Iopamidol are two of the more common non-ionic products being used today. Suggested dosages for Iohexol as a gastrointesinal contrast agent are as follows:

Cats:

Iohexol (240 mg I/ml concentration). Dilute the contrast medium 1:3 with water (1:2 if there is increased intraluminal fluid). Give at a dose of 10 ml/kg.

Williams J, Biller DS, Miyabayashi T, Leveille R. Evaluation of Iohexol as a gastrointestinal contrast medium in cats. Vet Radiol & Ultrasound 34:310-314, 1993.

Dogs:

Iohexol (300 mgI/ml concentration). Give at a dose of 700 mg I/kg with the Iohexol diluted with water to acheive a final volume of 10 ml/kg.

Agut A, Sanchez-Valverde MA, Lasaosa JM, Murciano J, Molina F. Use of Iohexol as a gastrointestinal contrast medium in the dog. Vet Radiol & Ultrasound 34:171-177, 1993.

Section 6

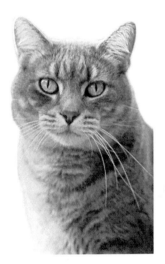

Urinary Tract

Selection of Appropriate Contrast Procedure

✓ For urinary bladder and urethra, use retrograde contrast procedures (cystography, urethrography).

✓ For kidneys and ureters, use excretory urography.

✓ Use history, physical examination, and laboratory data to determine affected area(s).

✓ Multiple areas may require making a cystogram, urethrogram, and excretory urogram.

☞ Remember that contrast radiography should always be preceded by survey radiography.

Contrast Examination of the Urinary Bladder (Cystography)

✓ Sedation is often helpful
✓ Use a flexible catheter for dogs
✓ Use a 3-way valve for control of contrast media

Indications

✓ Clinical signs such as dysuria, stranguria, hematuria, pyuria, incontinence

✓ Suspected cystitis, urinary bladder calculi, neoplasia

Positive Contrast Cystogram

✓ Ionic organic iodide

✓ This procedure is the best one for a possible ruptured urinary bladder.

✓ Dilute the organic iodine contrast medium 1:1 with sterile water.

✓ Infuse via urinary catheter until the bladder is moderately distended.

♥ Dosage: 5 ml/lb

💣 Individualize! Don't overfill the bladder!

✓ If you have a strong suspicion of rupture, give 20-30 ml, radiograph, and give additional contrast to distend the bladder if rupture is not apparent.

Negative Contrast Cystogram (Pneumocystogram)

✓ Air or carbon dioxide (CO_2) for negative and double contrast cystograms

> ✓ Air is cheaper and most convenient
>
> ✓ If the bladder mucosa is severely eroded, air may be forced into the blood stream and cause air embolism because of its high nitrogen content.
>
> ✓ CO_2 is a safer negative contrast because CO_2 is highly soluble in blood, and does not cause gas embolism.
>
> ✓ The incidence of air embolism from pneumocystography is very low. Most veterinarians use air. Avoid air if the bladder mucosa is severely damaged. There may be fewer problems if the animal is in left lateral recumbency since the air is more likely to be in the right side of the heart and will be pumped into the lungs.

✓ This is the least useful study.

✓ Can be used to detect urinary calculi

💣※ Can be misleading for evaluation of bladder wall thickness (Figure 6-1). What appears to be wall is wall + residual urine.

Double Contrast Cystogram

✓ Catheterize and empty the urinary bladder

✓ Instill 3-10 cc positive contrast (organic iodine contrast)

✓ Fill the bladder with air or CO_2, but watch for increased back pressure on syringe. (The bladder may not distend normally in animals with chronic cystitis.)

✓ Expose lateral, right ventrodorsal oblique, and left ventrodorsal oblique views.

✓ Oblique views avoid superimposition of vertebral column and bladder.

✓ You do not need to remove the contrast media after examination.

✓ This is the best general purpose contrast study.

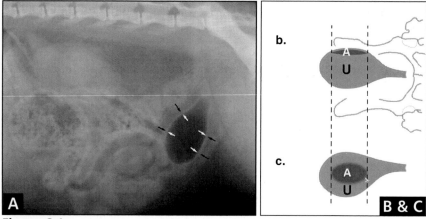

Figure 6-1

A. Normal negative contrast cystogram of a cat in lateral recumbancy. It is as though the observer is looking down on an air bubble in the bladder. The fluid opacity between the black arrows (serosal surface) and the white arrows is made up of bladder wall and residual urine and not just bladder wall. **B.** Diagram of a negative contrast cystogram exposed with the animal in lateral recumbency using a horizontal beam. Air (A) is shown as a black bubble positioned at the top of the urine (U) filled bladder. **C.** Diagram showing how the negative contrast study would appear if exposed using a vertical beam in the usual manner. Note that wall thickness cannot be determined. W=Wall.

Normal Double Contrast Cystogram

✔ Smooth walls

♥ A smooth central contrast puddle is seen (Figure 6-2A).

✔ Uniform wall thickness is 2-3 mm with a smooth mucosal border (Figures 6-2B and 6-2C)

Complications

✔ Tissue damage from catheterization.

✔ Iatrogenic infection resulting from catheterization.

✔ Air embolism is rare but can occur with severe mucosal damage.

💣 Over-distension can cause rupture especially if the wall is diseased.

Vesicoureteral Reflux

✔ Refers to reflux of urine from the urinary bladder into the ureters

✔ It can occur in normal animals.

✔ Negative or positive contrast is seen in the ureters and/or kidneys during positive or double contrast cystography (Figures 6-2D and 6-2E). ☉

♥ If it occurs in animals with cystitis, evaluate for ascending infection and pyelonephritis.

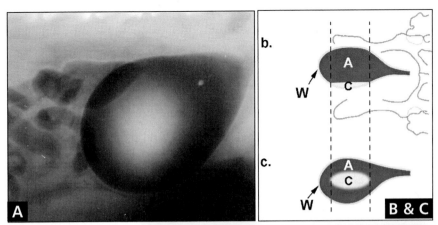

Figure 6-2

A. Lateral view of a normal double contrast cystogram in a dog. **B.** Diagram of a double contrast cystogram exposed with the animal in lateral recumbancy using a horizontal beam. Air (A) fills most of the urinary bladder. Contrast (C) forms a white puddle at the dependent side of the bladder and coats the wall (W) of the bladder. **C.** Diagram showing how the double contrast study would appear if exposed using a vertical beam in the usual manner. Note that the wall is visible. **D.** Double contrast cystogram in a cat showing vesicoureteral reflux of iodine contrast. The contrast agent can be seen in the renal pelvis and diverticula (arrow). **E.** Double contrast cystogram in a cat showing vesicoureteral reflux of

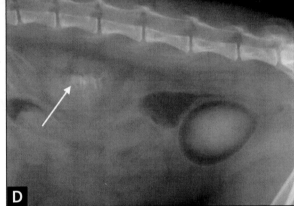

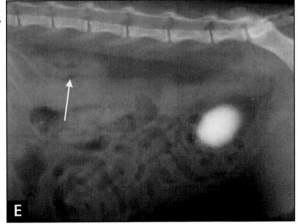

air. Air can be seen in the renal pelvis and diverticula (arrow).

Disorders of the Urinary Bladder

Urinary Calculi

Roentgen Signs on Survey Films

✓ Calculi that are radiopaque are usually composed of phosphate, oxalate, and silica.

✓ Calculi that are radiolucent are usually composed of cystine and urate.

✓ The radiographic appearance of urinary calculi is not a reliable indicator of composition.

✓ Differentiate other calcific opacities, e.g., dystrophic mineralization in neoplasms.

✓ Calculi can be solitary or multiple, small or large (Figure 6-3). ⊙

Roentgen Signs on Cystography

♥ The best procedure is double contrast cystogram (Figure 6-4A). ⊙

✓ Calculi are not as clearly seen in negative or positive contrast cystograms (Figure 6-4B).

✓ Calculi form filling defects in the central dependent portion of the contrast puddle.

✓ Margins are usually well-defined.

✓ Calculi may be irregularly shaped.

✓ You need to differentiate other filling defects (Figure 6-4C and Table 6-1) such as air bubbles, blood clots, and masses.

Ruptured Bladder

✓ Usually history of trauma

Roentgen Signs on Survey Films

♥ Variable loss of serosal detail depending on size and duration of tear (Figure 6-5A)

Roentgen Signs on Cystography

✓ A pneumocystogram is not recommended.

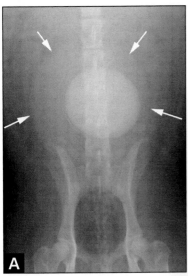

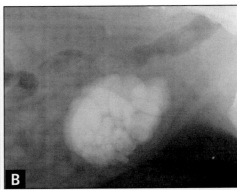

Figure 6-3

Calculi in the urinary bladder.
A. A large solitary calculus
(arrows indicate the margins
of the bladder wall). **B.** Multiple calculi in various sizes.
C. Multiple calculi are seen in
the bladder and prostatic
urethra. **D.** Further examination of the dog in Figure 6-
3C shows a large calculus at
the base of the os penis.
Arrows indicate the calculi.

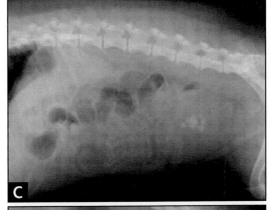

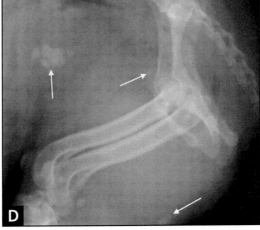

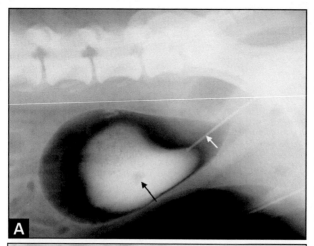

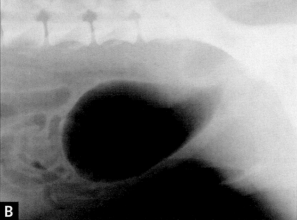

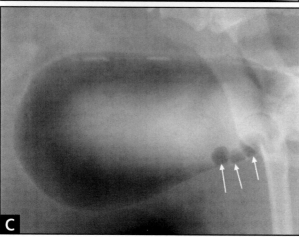

Figure 6-4
Cystography in a dog with multiple calculi. **A.** The calculi show as well-defined filling defects in a double contrast cystogram. The largest filling defect is likely a blood clot. White arrow:catheter. **B.** The calculi are not seen in a negative contrast cystogram. **C.** Air bubbles (arrows) may be seen as well-defined filling defects on the periphery of the contrast puddle and should not be confused with calculi.

Table 6-1
Filling Defects in Double Contrast Cystogram

Structure	Location	Margins	Shape	
Air bubbles	Periphery of the contrast "puddle".	Bright margin caused by the meniscus at the base of the bubble.	Circular	
Calculi	Central, dependent portion of the puddle.	Usually indistinct margins.	May be irregular	
Blood Cells	Center or periphery of contrast puddle. Free in lumen or attached to the mucosa.	Poorly marginated.	Irregular	
Masses	Variable but fixed.	Variable	Variable	

✔ A small amount of air leakage from the bladder after a pneumocystogram may be hard to differentiate from intraluminal GI gas.

☞ The procedure of choice is a positive contrast cystogram.

✔ The cystogram portion of an excretory urogram can also be used as it can help differentiate a ruptured bladder from ruptured ureter.

♥ Positive contrast can be seen free in the abdominal cavity outlining serosal surfaces (Figure 6-5B).

✔ Sometimes the bladder wall is not completely ruptured, but the mucosa protrudes through torn muscle and serosal layers (Figure 6-6).

Cystitis

Roentgen Signs on Survey Films

✔ No signs are seen unless gas or dystrophic mineralization is present.

Roentgen Signs on Cystography

✔ Use a double-contrast cystogram to assess bladder wall thickness and mucosa.

Acute cystitis:

  ✔ The wall is normal or only slightly thickened.

Chronic cystitis (Figure 6-7):

  ✔ Wall is thickened uniformly or in focal areas. ⊙

  ✔ Mucosa is frequently irregular.

  ✔ There may be mucosal ulceration or diverticula.

Severe chronic cystitis:

  ✔ May resemble infiltrating bladder neoplasia.

  ✔ Bladder wall may be thickened, fibrotic, and is no longer distensible.

  ✔ Vesicoureteral reflux will occur after injection of only a small amount of contrast.

Emphysematous Cystitis

✔ Gas is in the wall, ligaments, or lumen of the urinary bladder

✔ Usually associated with diabetes mellitus: glucose-fermenting bacteria produce gas

✔ May see gas produced by clostridial organisms.

✔ Gas may be iatrogenic due to catheterization or cystocentesis.

Figure 6-5

A. Note the loss of serosal detail in this dog that was hit by a car. Barium is seen in the colon from a previous procedure. **B.** An excretory urogram was performed. Positive contrast is leaking into the peritoneal cavity. Serosal surfaces are visible because of the contrast within the peritoneum.

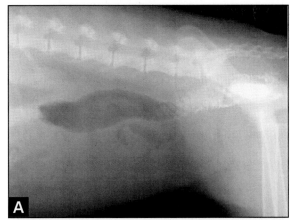

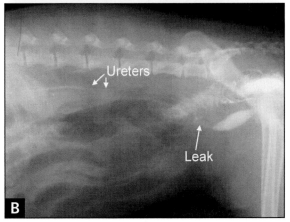

Figure 6-6

A positive contrast cystogram shows a mucosal hernia (arrows) in this dog with a history of trauma.

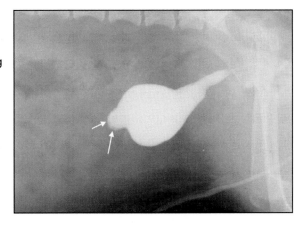

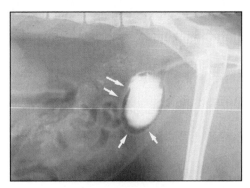

Figure 6-7
Double contrast cystogram in a cat with chronic cystitis causing thickening of the dorsal urinary bladder wall. Arrows indicate the serosal surface of the bladder. Notice that the contrast puddle is too large; the amount of contrast needed was overestimated.

Roentgen Signs on Survey Films

♥ Gas is visible in the wall, ligaments, or lumen (Figure 6-8) ⊙

Roentgen Signs on Cystography

✓ A double contrast cystogram could be made for further evaluation of the wall

✓ Changes would be as for cystitis without gas.

Urinary Bladder Neoplasia

✓ Often have history of hematuria

✓ Most common type is transitional cell carcinoma

✓ Common site is at the urinary trigone although other areas can be affected

♥ Consider implications for the kidneys if a mass is present at the trigone (see Disorders of the Kidneys)

✓ Remember to expose the thoracic films to check for pulmonary metastasis

Roentgen Signs on Survey Films

✓ Usually appears normal

✓ May see mineralization in the tumer

Roentgen Signs on Cystography

✓ A double contrast cystogram is the procedure of choice (Figure 6-9)

✓ Expose right lateral, left lateral, left ventrodorsal oblique, and right ventrodorsal oblique views.

♥ Filling defect is seen when a mass is on the dependent side protruding into the contrast puddle.

Figure 6-8
Lateral view of the caudal abdomen of a dog. Although it appears that a negative contrast cystogram was performed, the air in the bladder lumen was the result of emphysematous cystitis secondary to diabetes mellitus.

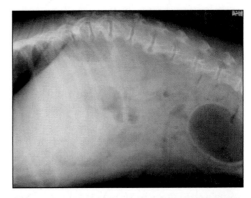

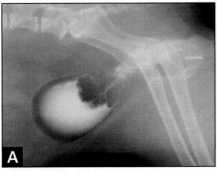

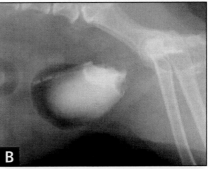

Figure 6-9
Double contrast cystogram in a dog with transitional cell carcinoma. **A.** Left lateral recumbent view: the mass appears as a filling defect when it is on the dependent side of the urinary bladder. **B.** Right lateral recumbent view: the mass is coated with contrast and is opaque when it is on the non-dependent side of the bladder. **C.** Ventrodorsal view: the mass shows as a filling defect on the left side of the bladder.

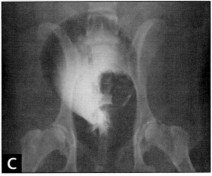

♥ The mass is coated with contrast when it is on the non-dependent side of the bladder and surrounded by air.

Contrast Examination of the Urethra (Urethrography)

✓ Urethral disorders are more common in males

Indications

✓ Clinical signs include dysuria, stranguria, hematuria, incontinence

✓ Contrast procedure of choice to assess the urethral lumen and mucosa to diagnose, localize, and determine extent and severity of urethral neoplasia, inflammatory lesions, or calculi

Technique

✓ A lateral survey of the caudal abdomen shows the proximal urethra

✓ Survey with the rear limbs pulled cranially and dorsally over the abdomen to allow visualization of the urethral arch and distal urethra without superimposition of rear limbs

✓ Use sedation

✓ Catheterize with a small (6 French) Foley catheter

✓ Fill the catheter with fluid to avoid introducing air bubbles. (Bubbles may be hard to differentiate from radiolucent calculi).

✓ Catheter has small inflatable cuff near the tip; place tip in distal urethra. (Second injection can be made with tip at pelvic brim.)

✓ Inflate the cuff to lock the catheter in the penis.

✓ Inject 2-3 ml of 2% lidocaine diluted 1:1 with sterile water into the urethra to prevent pain and spasm of the urethra.

✓ Inject 5-15 ml contrast rapidly 1-2 minutes later.

✓ Expose the lateral radiograph during the injection with legs pulled cranially and dorsally over the abdomen. Have the cassette in place and start the rotor of the x-ray machine at the beginning of injection. The urethra is mildly dilated during the radiographic exposure, allowing optimal visualization of the urethral lumen.

✓ Immediately expose slightly oblique ventrodorsal view.

Normal Urethrogram

♥ Urethra should be smooth and filled with contrast (Figure 6-10)

✓ Urethra narrows normally as it passes through the prostate gland.

Disorders of the Urethra

Urethral Calculi

Roentgen Signs on Survey Films

✓ Radiopaque calculi are visible in the urethra and urinary bladder

✓ The most common location is at the caudal aspect of the os penis (Figure 6-11) ⊙

✓ Occasionally, unusual foreign bodies are seen (Figure 6-12A).

Figure 6-10
Normal urethrogram of a male dog.

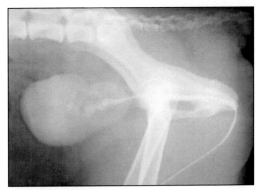

Figure 6-11
An 11- year old male Dachshund with urethral calculi. **A.** Lateral survey radiograph of the urethra shows 3 calculi at the proximal end of the os penis (arrow). **B.** Ventrodorsal view. **C.** Lateral urethrogram shows filling defects in the contrast column caused by urethral calculi (C). The tip (T) of the catheter is visible distally.

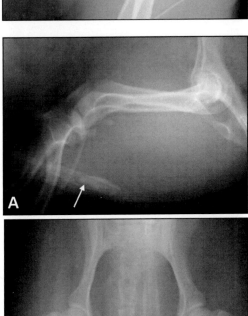

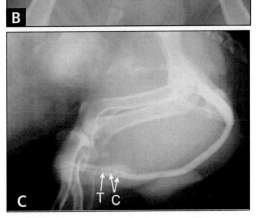

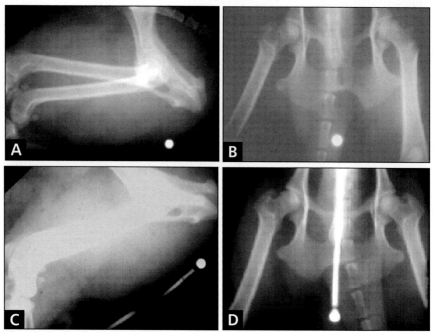

Figure 6-12
Survey radiographs of the urethra of a male dog that was shot. Is gunshot really in the urethra? **A.** Lateral view. **B.** Ventrodorsal view. A urethrogram confirmed that gunshot was in the urethra. Iodine contrast is in the urethra distal to the gunshot. **C.** Lateral urethrogram. **D.** Ventrodorsal urethrogram.

Roentgen Signs on Retrograde Urethrogram

Filling Defects

✓ Distinguish between calculi, air bubbles, and blood clots (Table 6-2).

✓ Blood clots may come from the urinary bladder, traumatized urethral tissue, or proliferative mucosal disease associated with trauma, neoplasia, or urethral infection.

✓ Contrast can be used to determine if the foreign material seen on survey films is present in the urethra (Figure 6-12B).

✓ Urethral infection and urolithiasis can cause painful reflex spasms of the urethra

    Spasms may be seen as marked luminal narrowing

    Distinguish urethral spasm and stricture by infusing dilute lidocaine into the lumen

    Spasms will be relieved, and strictures will be unchanged

Table 6-2
Filling Defects in Urethrogram

Structure	Location In Lumen	Effect On Lumen	Margins	Shape
Air bubbles	Symmetrically placed	No distension	Smooth, distinct	Round
Blood clots	Asymmetrically placed	No distension	Irregular, indistinct	Irregular
Calculi	Asymmetrically placed	Distension if large	Irregular, indistinct	Irregular
Mass (neoplasia, scar tissue)	Asymmetrically placed	Pushes inward	Variable	Usually irregular

Obstructive Uropathy

✔ Indentify obstructing calculi, masses, or anomalies.

✔ Evaluate the bladder wall thickness and irregularity

✔ Define the presence or extent of urethral strictures

✔ Determine if renal involvement is unilateral or bilateral

✔ Serial radiographic examinations evaluate progression of disease or response to treatment

💣※ Remember that obstructive uropathy can occur at a higher level (bladder or ureter).

Ruptured Urethra

Roentgen Signs on Survey Films

✔ May be increased opacity in the pelvic canal and caudoventral abdomen

✔ May be loss of serosal detail if urine is in the peritoneal cavity

✔ May be associated pelvic fractures

Roentgen Signs on Retrograde Urethrography

✔ Positive contrast can be seen in the periurethral tissues (Figure 6-13).

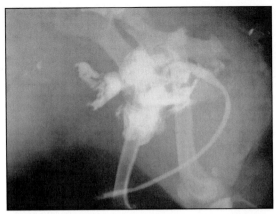

Figure 6-13
Lateral urethrogram of a male Peke-A-Poo who was hit by a car and sustained a fractured pelvis. Rupture of the urethra is apparent.

Contrast Examination of the Kidneys and Ureters–Excretory Urogram

✓ Also known as intravenous urogram (IVU) or intravenous pyelogram (IVP)

Indications

✓ Clinical signs such as polyuria, polydipsia, anuria, hematuria, inappropriate urination

✓ Elevated blood chemistries (BUN, creatinine)

✓ Diseases which can be diagnosed include hydronephrosis, hydroureter, pyelonephritis, ectopic ureter, and renal calculi.

✓ Excretory urography is useful whenever there is a need to see the renal parenchyma, pelvis, or ureters.

✓ Contrast study is also useful for bladder disease when catheterization is not possible

Selection of Contrast Agent

✓ Use a sterile water soluble iodine product.

✓ Nonionic iodine products have fewer side effects.

✓ Nausea and retching after rapid IV administration of organic iodine contrast is not uncommon, especially in cats.

✓ Severe anaphylactoid reactions are rare.

✓ Organic iodine media can be used safely even in uremic animals.

Technique

✓ Fast the animal for 24 hours before taking urinary contrast studies.

✓ Cleansing enemas should be administered 1-2 hours before.

✓ Withhold water for 6-12 hours before if that is possible. Do not withhold water if the animal is uremic or dehydrated. Withholding will cause renal resorption of fluid and enhance concentration of contrast medium in urine.

✓ Survey radiographs to evaluate preparation, possibly give additional information, and get a baseline.

✓ Indwelling catheter in the cephalic vein

Facilitate the injection of large volume of contrast medium

Reduce the likelihood of causing a perivascular injection

Contrast media are irritating, and may cause discomfort and tissue necrosis if injected perivascularily

Provide a central line for drug administration in case of hypovolemic shock

✓ You can use abdominal compression to obstruct the flow, and to distend renal pelves and proximal ureters.

Place a tight bandage around the abdomen just cranial to the pubis

Place the animal in dorsal recumbency and extend a compression band across the x-ray table

Sedation may be needed

Iodine Dose

♥ 600-800 mg iodine/kg given intravenously

✓ Give in 1-2 minutes

✓ Iodine is excreted mainly by glomerular filtration (less than 1% excretion by liver and small bowel) in normal animals.

Sequence of Films

Ventro-dorsal	Lateral	Oblique
Immediate		
5 minutes	5 minutes	5 minutes for ureteral termination
20 minutes		
40 minutes		

If renal pelves and ureters are well defined, remove compression after 20 minute films. Expose ventrodorsal and lateral films 5 minutes after release.

Normal Excretory Urogram

Arteriogram Phase ◉

✓ During or immediately after injections of contrast

✓ Usually you don't see this phase

✓ Contrast is briefly in the arteries and arterioles (Figure 6-14)

✓ Early nephrogram is present

Nephrogram Phase

✓ Immediate (Figure 6-15) – contrast is in renal parenchyma, as the kidneys are more radiopaque

✓ Starts 7-10 seconds after injection of contrast

✓ The best contrast is at 10-20 seconds

✓ Progressive fading occurs in 1-3 hours

✓ This phase is caused by contrast in the proximal renal tubules.

✓ Opacity depends on contrast dose, glomerular filtration rate, and renal tubular osmolarity.

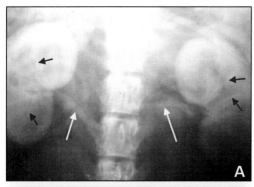
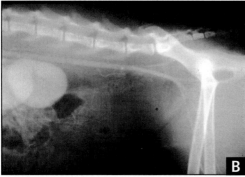

Figure 6-14
Lateral excretory urogram showing the arteriogram phase. Contrast is seen in the renal arteries (white arrows and their branches (black arrows). An early nephrogram is present

Figure 6-15

Ventrodorsal excretory urogram shows the nephrogram phase immediately after injection of contrast. Notice that contrast is not yet in the renal pelvis.

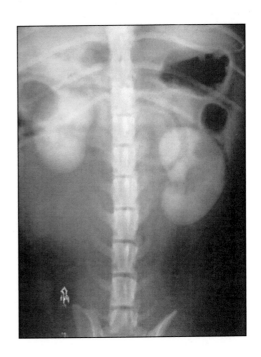

Pyelogram Phase (Figure 6-16A)

✓ It is much more distinct when compression is applied (Figure 6-16B) ⊙

✓ Starts 1-3 minutes after injection

✓ The best contrast is in the first 20 minutes

✓ It is caused by the contrast in the renal diverticula, pelves, and ureters

✓ Opacity depends on concentration of contrast in the urine and the volume of urine in the collecting system

✓ Diverticula have a width of less than 1-2 mm without compression

✓ Proximal ureter has a width less than 2-3 mm without compression

✓ Uremic patients may take 20-40 minutes or longer for their renal pelves to fill.

✓ In ureteral peristalsis, ureters appear discontinuous because of peristaltic waves.

Cystogram Phase

✓ Contrast in urinary bladder (Figures 6-17A and 6-17B). ⊙

✓ Be careful of artifact when the bladder is incompletely filled.

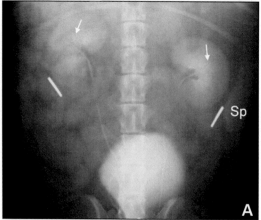

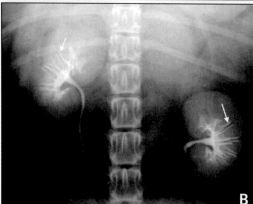

Figure 6-16
Ventrodorsal excretory urogram shows the pyelogram phase. **A.** Without compression 10 minutes after injection. Diverticula are only faintly visualized (arrows). Ovario-hysterectomy clamps are seen caudal to the kidneys. Sp:Spleen. **B.** With compression at 5 minutes as seen in another dog. Diverticula are now clearly seen.

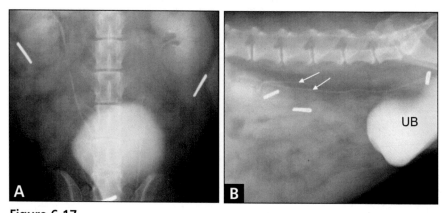

Figure 6-17
Excretory urogram shows the cystogram phase. Notice that the nephrogram and pyelogram phases are also present. Arrows: ureters, UB: urinary bladder. **A.** Ventrodorsal view. **B.** Lateral view.

Complications
✓ Vomiting (especially in cats)

✓ Dehydration with ionic iodine products

✓ Pulmonary edema

✓ Allergic reaction (more common in people)

💣※ Contrast-induced acute tubular nephrosis -
   Persistent nephrogram, no pyelogram
   Start intravenous fluids and diuretics

Disorders of the Kidneys and Ureters

Chronic Renal Disease
Chronic interstitial or glomerular nephritis

Roentgen Signs on Survey Films
Kidneys may be small (Figures 6-18A and 6-18B)

Kidneys may be irregular

Renal Dysplasia
✓ Appearance of renal dysplasia is similar to that of chronic interstitial or glomerular nephritis: small, sometimes irregular kidneys (Figure 6-18C). ⊙

✓ Kidneys fail to develop properly.

✓ Blood creatinine and urea nitrogen levels are often surprisingly high in animals that don't look that sick.

✓ It can be familial in some breeds.

Transitional Cell Carcinoma of the Urinary Bladder

Implications for the Kidneys
✓ There may be no change

✓ It can cause hydronephrosis and hydroureter if the bladder mass obstructs the ureters.

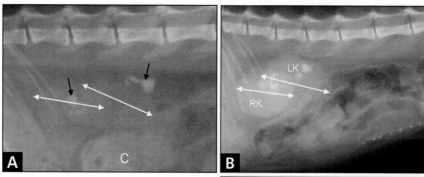

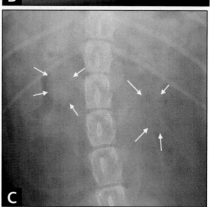

Figure 6-18
A. Chronic renal disease in a 6-year old cat. Calculi (black arrows) were in the renal pelves. The kidneys (white double-headed arrows) were small and irregular. Radiopaque fecal material in the colon (C) was attributed to dehydration secondary to renal failure. **B.** Lateral excretory urogram 30 minutes after the injection of contrast shows the small, irregular kidneys. A normal pyelogram was never seen on either side because of partial obstruction caused by the calculi.
(Courtesy of Northlake Veterinary Specialists, Clarkson, GA.) **C.** Ventrodorsal radiograph of a 1-year old dog shows abnormally small and malformed kidneys (arrows) secondary to renal dysplasia.

Hydronephrosis

✓ Dilation of the renal pelvis and diverticula

✓ Occurs secondary to partial or complete obstruction (e.g., neoplasia at bladder trigone, ectopic ureter, ureteral calculus).

✓ In severe cases, the kidney can literally become a bag of urine.

Roentgen Signs on Survey Films

✓ Kidneys may be normal or enlarged

Roentgen Signs on Excretory Urography

♥ Dilatation of the renal pelves and diverticula (Figure 6-19). ⊙

✓ Diverticula are sharp

✓ Ureters may also be dilated (hydroureter)

✓ In severe cases, a thin rim of functional tissue may opacify and surround the dilated collecting system.

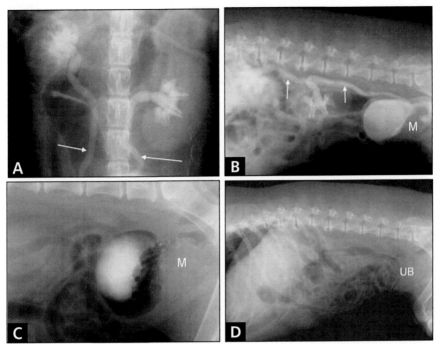

Figure 6-19
Excretory urogram of 13-year old Basset Hound shows bilateral hydronephrosis and hydroureter (arrows) secondary to transitional cell carcinoma in the urinary bladder. **A.** Ventrodorsal view. **B.** Lateral view. M:mass in the urinary bladder. **C.** Lateral cystogram also shows a mass (M) at the trigone. Histopathology showed transitional cell carcinoma. **D.** The survey radiography does not indicate any problem. UB:urinary bladder.

Renal Calculi

Roentgen Signs on Survey Films

✓ Many are radiopaque (Figure 6-20A)

✓ Not all calcific renal opacities represent calculi

✓ Differentiate nephrocalcinosis (dystrophic calcification of infarcts, tumors, other lesions)

Roentgen Signs on Excretory Urography

☞ **Radiopacity is relative!**

✓ Both radiolucent and radiopaque calculi appear as well marginated filling defects (Figure 6-20B)

♥ Nephrocalcinosis does not cause a filling defect.

✓ Remember to assess the pelvis and ureter for dilatation.

💣※ Blood clots and chronic pyelonephritis can also cause filling defects.

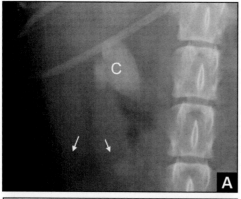

Figure 6-20
A. Survey radiograph shows a radiopaque renal calculus (C). The right kidney is not clearly seen but margins of the caudal pole are visible (arrows). **B.** The calculus shows as a filling defect in the contrast-filled renal pelvis when excretory urography was performed. (The calculus is more opaque than renal tissue but less opaque than iodine contrast.)

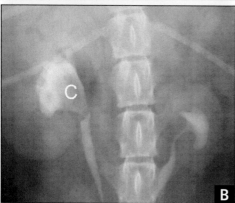

Pyelonephritis

Acute Pyelonephritis

Roentgen Signs on Survey Films

✓ Survey radiographs may be normal

✓ Clinically increased kidney size has been reported but enlarged kidneys were not seen in controlled studies on induced pyelonephritis.

Roentgen Signs on Excretory Urography

✓ Decreased opacity of the nephrogram

✓ Delayed filling of the pyelogram

✓ Dilatation of the renal pelvis and proximal ureters

♥ If the pelvis is dilated, the diverticula are usually absent or blunted

♥ May distinguish between pyelonephritis and obstruction

Acute obstructive uropathy: pelvis and diverticula are distended

(With severe hydronephrosis, pelvis and diverticula may be indistinguishable)

Pyelonephritis: Pelvis may be distended with absence of diverticular filling.

If pelvic distention is severe, the collecting system may be nonvisualized.

✓ Kidney may appear normal

Chronic Pyelonephritis
Roentgen Signs on Survey Films

✓ Survey radiographs may be normal.

✓ In chronic disease, may see "end-stage" kidneys

Kidneys are small

Capsule is irregular

The signs are not specific for pyelonephritis

✓ Pyelonephritis may be suggested by the presence of predisposing causes, e.g., uroliths, ureteral ectopia, vesicoureteral reflux.

Roentgen Signs on Excretory Urography

♥ Kidneys are usually reduced in size.

♥ Dilatation and irregularity of the renal pelvis is seen from scarring and scar retraction (Figure 6-21).

✓ Filling defects within the renal pelvis are caused by cellular debris, blood clots, or uroliths.

✓ Dilatation of the proximal ureters

✓ Kidney may be normal

Note:

💣※ With an irregular pelvis +/- filling defects, the differential must include neoplasia.

Renal Neoplasia
Roentgen Signs on Survey Films

✓ May be normal; may be enlarged or deformed

♥ Lymphosarcoma usually causes uniform enlargement.

♥ Adenocarcinoma is more likely to present as a mass deforming the kidney.

Roentgen Signs on Excretory Urography

✓ May be an area of non-contrast in the nephrogram

✓ Distortion or deviation of the pelvis/diverticula (Figure 6-22).

✓ Dilatation of the diverticula, pelves, or ureters

✓ May appear normal

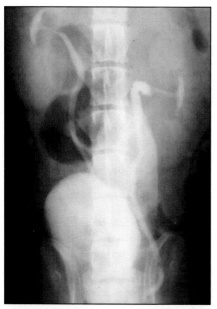

Figure 6-21
Excretory urogram of a dog with chronic pyelonephritis. Notice blunting of the pelvic diverticula, filling defects, and hydroureter.

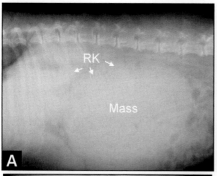

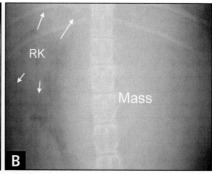

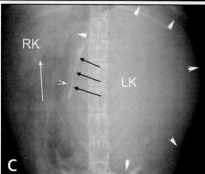

Figure 6-22
A large mass is in the abdomen of this Miniature Poodle. A normal left kidney cannot be seen separately from the mass. RK: right kidney. **A.** Lateral view. **B.** Ventrodorsal view. **C.** Ventrodorsal excretory urogram. The right renal pelvis (white arrows) is normal but the mass in the left kidney is compressing the left renal pelvis (black arrows). White arrowheads indicate the margins of the neoplastic left kidney. LK: left kidney.

Polycystic Renal Disease

✓ Small renal cysts are frequently seen with ultrasonography without causing clinical signs and without altering the renal silhouette on radiographs.

✓ In "polycystic renal disease," a significant amount of renal tubules are replaced by cysts.

✓ Disease occurs in young dogs and cats (renal dysplasia).

Roentgen Signs on Survey Films

✓ Kidneys may appear normal.

✓ Kidneys may be enlarged or distorted (Figure 6-23). ⊙

Roentgen Signs on Excretory Urography

♥ Filling defects in the nephrogram indicate the location of cysts.

Perirenal Pseudocyst

✓ Can be unilateral or bilateral (Figure 6-24).

✓ Transudate or modified transudate collects between the renal capsule and parenchyma because of chronic renal disease.

✓ Surgical resection of the capsule is necessary to stop fluid formation.

✓ Renal disease progresses in spite of resection.

✓ Prognosis depends on the severity of renal disease, which is ultimately fatal.

✓ In one study, cats survived a median of 9 months after capsular resection.

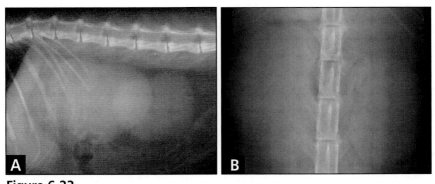

Figure 6-23
A. Lateral survey film of the abdomen of a 4 year old cat with polycystic renal disease. **B.** Ventrodorsal view shows the enlarged kidneys.

Roentgen Signs on Survey Films

✓ Enlarged renal shadow or fluid-opaque mass

✓ Mass begins dorsally but can extend to the abdominal floor.

☛ Key sign is nonvisualization of the kidney on the same side as the mass (Figure 6-24A).

Roentgen Signs on Excretory Urography

♥ Nephrogram is seen within the fluid opaque mass (Figure 6-24B). ☉

♥ The kidneys are frequently small and irregular.

Compensatory Hypertrophy

✓ A kidney enlarges to compensate for disease in the other kidney, or a missing kidney

Roentgen Signs on Survey Films

✓ One kidney is small or missing; the other is enlarged.

Roentgen Signs on Excretory Urography

✓ Hypertrophied kidney is otherwise normal.

Functional Evaluation of the Kidney

✓ The excretory urogram is only a crude indication of renal function.

✓ Absence of a nephrogram can be due to renal or nonrenal disease, usually cardiac disease.

☛ Remember that the nephrogram can be normal even when renal disease is severe.

♥ Presence of only one nephrogram suggests a missing or nonfunctional kidney or obstruction (Figure 6-25).

☛ However, a normal nephrogram does not ensure good renal function.

♥ Additional function studies (e.g., nuclear scintigraphy) should be performed.

💣 Never remove a kidney unless you are sure the remaining kidney is functional.

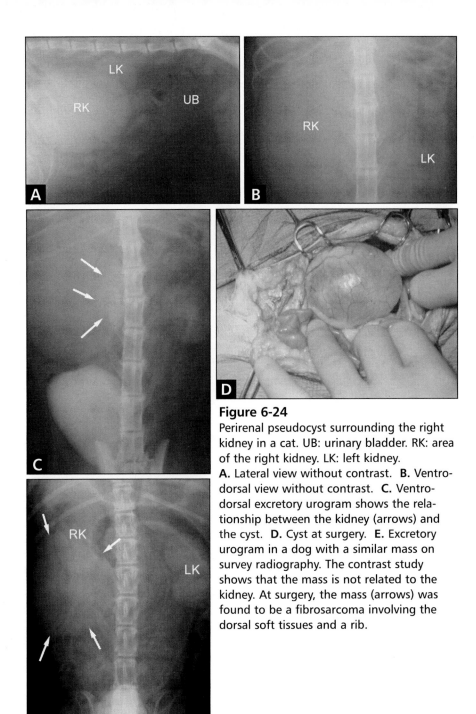

Figure 6-24

Perirenal pseudocyst surrounding the right kidney in a cat. UB: urinary bladder. RK: area of the right kidney. LK: left kidney. **A.** Lateral view without contrast. **B.** Ventrodorsal view without contrast. **C.** Ventrodorsal excretory urogram shows the relationship between the kidney (arrows) and the cyst. **D.** Cyst at surgery. **E.** Excretory urogram in a dog with a similar mass on survey radiography. The contrast study shows that the mass is not related to the kidney. At surgery, the mass (arrows) was found to be a fibrosarcoma involving the dorsal soft tissues and a rib.

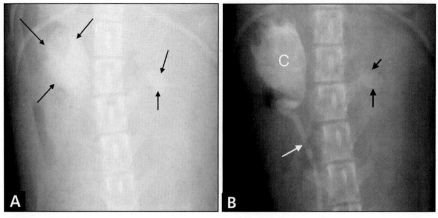

Figure 6-25
A. Survey radiographs of the abdomen of a 2-year old Yorkshire Terrier shows a calculi in both kidneys (arrows). **B.** Excretory urography was performed. Contrast is seen in the right renal pelvis and ureter (white arrow). The large calculus (C) in the right kidney causes a filling defect in the contrast in the renal pelvis. The calculus (black arrows) in the left kidney is smaller, but there is no excretion of contrast into the left renal pelvis and ureter suggesting the left kidney is non-functional.

Ruptured Ureter

Roentgen Signs on Survey Films

✓ Loss of detail in the retroperitoneal space.

✓ Retroperitoneal space is fluid-opaque with normal fat not visible.

✓ Increased size of the retroperitoneal space.

Roentgen Signs on Excretory Urography

♥ Positive contrast is seen in the retroperitoneal space outside the ureter (Figure 6-26).

✓ Rupture of the ureter can lead to periureteral inflammaion and ureteral ileus.

Ureteral Ileus

☞ Remember ureters display peristalsis and radiographs are made at one point at time.

☞ Peristalsis causes the ureters to normally appear discontinuous.

✓ Ileus can occur with inflammation, trauma, and obstruction.

✓ Ileus can be seen with hydronephrosis.

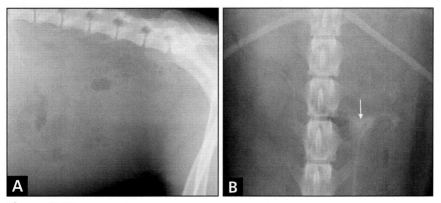

Figure 6-26
Mixed-breed female dog hit by a car the night before radiography. **A.** Survey radiographs show poor serosal detail and increased fluid opacity in the retroperitoneal space. **B.** Excretory urography confirms rupture of the ureter into the retroperitoneal space (arrow).

Roentgen Signs on Survey Films

✓ Ureter(s) may appear enlarged.

Roentgen Signs on Excretory Urography

✓ May be signs of trauma

♥ A ureter with ileus appears as a continuous column of contrast (Figure 6-27).

✓ There may be variable dilation

Figure 6-27
Excretory urogram of a dog with a ruptured ureter and ileus in other ureter. The dog was hit by a car.

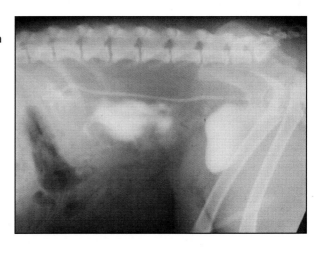

Ureteral Calculi

Roentgen Signs on Survey Films

✔ Small radiopacities may be in the retroperitoneal space (Figure 6-28A). ⊙

✔ May be able to see with ultrasound

💣※ Differentiate:

> Deep circumflex iliac arteries seen in the end-on projection (Figure 6-28D)

> Superimposition of nipples in the caudal abdomen (can "paint" nipples with barium and expose another film)

> Extraneous material in the intestine

Roentgen Signs on Excretory Urography

♥ Filling defect in contrast column in ureter (Figure 6-28C)

♥ Ureter dilated proximal to obstruction

Primary Ureteritis

Is uncommon

Roentgen Signs on Survey Films

Usually appears normal

Roentgen Signs on Excretory Urography

✔ Irregularity of the urothelium

✔ Ureteral ileus

✔ Signs are nonspecific

✔ Radiographic assessment based on the presence of conditions known to predispose ureteral infection such as calculi, vesicoureteral reflux, and ureteral ectopia.

✔ Ureteral ileus and distension are common and normal after any ureteral surgery

> Appear unrelated to infection

> Usually resolve after several weeks

Ectopic Ureter

✔ Ureter enters the urethra rather than the urinary bladder.

✔ The ureter may appear to connect to the bladder but may tunnel through the wall of the bladder to terminate in the urethra.

Figure 6-28

Calculus in the right ureter of a cat. RK:right kidney; LK:left kidney. **A.** Lateral survey radiograph shows a small opacity (white arrow) caudal to the kidneys (K). **B.** Ventrodorsal view shows the opacity (white arrow) at the caudal pole of the right kidney. White arrowheads mark the margins of the kidneys. **C.** Ventrodorsal excretory urogram at 40 minutes shows dilation of the right renal pelvis and the right ureter proximal to the calculus (white arrow). A normal pyelogram was never seen in the smaller left kidney, causing concern for the functional status of the kidney.

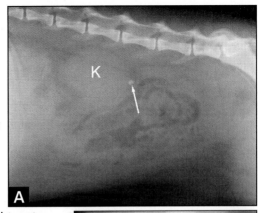

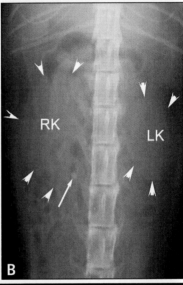

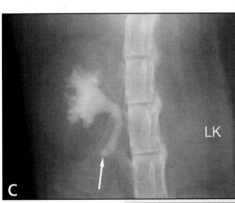

D. Lateral arteriogram in a dog shows the location of the circumflex iliac artery (arrow), which can be mistaken for a ureteral calculus when viewed end-on.

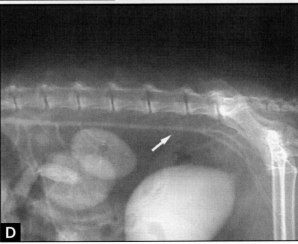

Roentgen Signs on Survey Films

Usually none

Roentgen Signs on Excretory Urography

✓ The signs can be difficult to see.

✓ Air in the bladder can help you see where ureters enter.

✓ Oblique views may be helpful.

♥ The ureter may by-pass the urinary bladder (Figure 6-29).

✓ Contrast may be visible in the urethra and/or vagina.

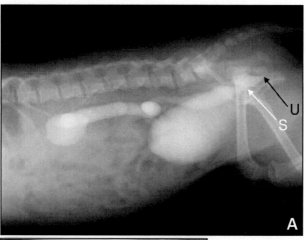

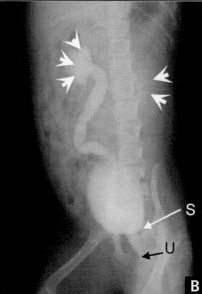

Figure 6-29
Excretory urogram shows an ectopic ureter in a 4-year old Poodle. U: entry of the ectopic ureter into the urethra, S: approximate location of the bladder sphincter. **A.** Lateral view. **B.** Ventro-dorsal view to allow better visualization of the entry of the right ureter into the urethra. Short white arrows indicate the dilated right renal pelvis and the normal diverticula of the left renal pelvis.

Section 7

Reproductive Tract

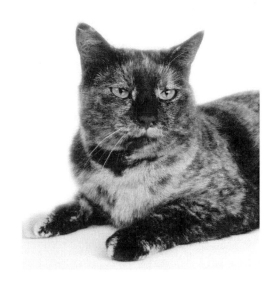

Female: Uterus and Ovaries

✓ Normal ovaries and the normal nongravid uterus are not identified as distinct structures in survey films.

Pregnancy

Roentgen Signs

⌐ The uterus will not be visible until it becomes larger than intestinal loops.

♥ Enlarged tortuous loops are the earliest sign of uterine enlargement.

✓ Significant fetal mineralization does not occur until about the 42nd day of pregnancy (Figure 7-1).

✓ Later skeletal heads and spines become apparent.

✓ Although ultrasonography can be used to diagnose pregnancy at an early stage, radiography is more accurate for determination of the number of fetuses.

Disorders of the Female Reproductive Tract

Pyometra and Other Causes of Uterine Enlargement

Roentgen Signs

♥ Tortuous tubular structures are most visible on the lateral view (see Figure 4-18).

✓ Rarely, localized enlargement of a small segment of the uterus will be seen (Figure 7-2). ⊙

✓ A wooden spoon or commercially available paddle can be used to isolate the uterus (Figure 7-3). ⊙

💣 Remember that radiographs show only an enlarged uterus.

Figure 7-1
A. Lateral radiograph of a pregnant dog at 42 days gestation. Fetal skeletons are barely visible (white arrows). Black arrows indicate the margins of a enlarged uterine horn. **B.** Close-up lateral view. H: head, S: spine. **C.** At 47 days, the heads (H) and spines (S) are more visible.

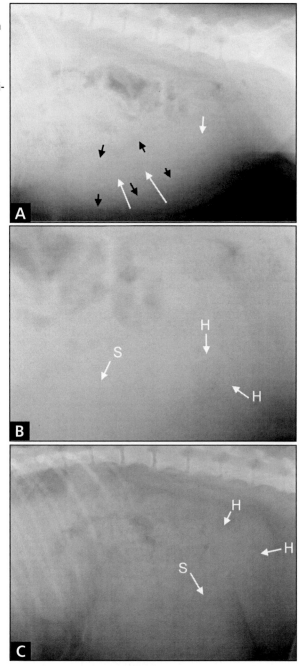

✓ History and other diagnostic procedures (physical examination, ultrasound, blood tests) should be used to differentiate other causes of uterine enlargement such as pregnancy, mucometra, and neoplasia.

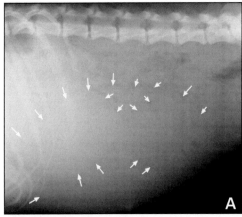

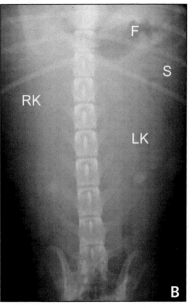

Figure 7-2
Lateral radiograph of a dog with pyometra localized to the tip of one horn. The diseased uterus could easily be confused with a splenic mass but, the tubular nature can be seen if the mass is closely examined. **A.** Lateral view. Arrows indicate various margins of the uterine horn. **B.** Ventrodorsal view. The mass occupies most of the mid-abdomen. The right (RK) and left (LK) kidneys can be seen superimposed over the mass. F: fundus; S: spleen.

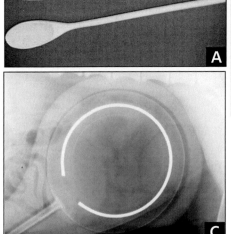

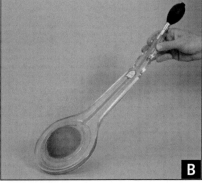

Figure 7-3
A. Wooden spoons used to isolate the uterus to confirm pyometra.
B. Commercial paddle. **C.** Uterus (with pyometra) isolated between the colon and urinary bladder using a commercial paddle to push the intestines away.

Dystocia

✓ The cause of dystocia is frequently not radiographically apparent.

Roentgen Signs

✓ The fetus may be too large compared to maternal pelvis (Figure 7-4).

✓ Radiography may be used to confirm that a retained fetus is present.

✓ Look for signs of fetal death.

Fetal Death

Roentgen Signs

✓ Loss of fetal flexion

✓ Gas in the uterus, in the fetal thoracic or abdominal cavities, or in fetal vessels (Figure 7-5).

✓ Collapse of the skull so that the bones overlap

✓ Mummified fetus appears as a mineralized mass in which fetal bones appear compressed and barely recognizable.

Figure 7-4
Lateral view of a dog with a fetus too large for the pelvic canal.

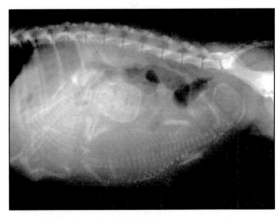

Ovarian Neoplasia

Roentgen Signs

♥ Ovarian ligaments stretch to allow enlarged ovaries to descend to the abdominal floor.

✓ Surrounding intestinal loops are pushed medially. See page 54 for additional details.

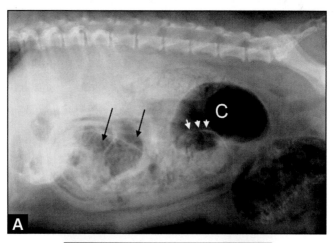

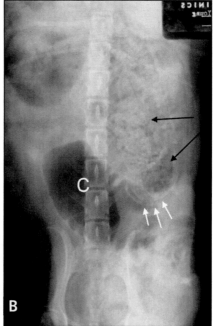

Figure 7-5
Radiographs of a pregnant dog. Gas in the uterus and fetal cavities (black arrows) and overlapping of bones of the skull (white arrows) indicates fetal death. C:colon. **A.** Lateral view. **B.** Ventrodorsal view.

Disorders of the Male Reproductive Tract

Retained Testicles and Prostate Gland

✓ Retained testicles are found anywhere between the caudal aspect of the kidneys and the inguinal ring.

✓ Nondiseased retained testicles are not likely to be seen radiographically.

✓ The prostate gland is located at the neck of the urinary bladder and is in the pelvic canal in young and neutered males.

✓ The prostate gland may be visible caudal to the urinary bladder on the abdominal floor in older intact males.

Testicular Masses

✓ Retained testicles are more likely to become neoplastic or cystic than normally descended scrotal testicles.

Roentgen Signs

♥ Midabdominal mass is located on the floor of the abdomen (Figure 7-6). ☉

✓ Cranial, dorsal, and caudal displacement of the intestines is seen.

💣※ Differentiate a splenic mass, mesenteric/enteric mass, and pedunculated hepatic mass.

Prostatic Enlargement

✓ Most common differentials are benign prostatic hyperplasia, prostatitis, neoplasia, and prostatic or paraprostatic cysts or abscesses.

✓ Recognize that the urinary bladder and enlarged prostate gland both present as fluid opacities in the caudoventral abdomen.

💣※ A solitary fluid opacity is most likely the urinary bladder but could be the prostate gland if the bladder is empty.

♥ Cystography could be performed to identify the bladder if necessary (see Figure 4-17).

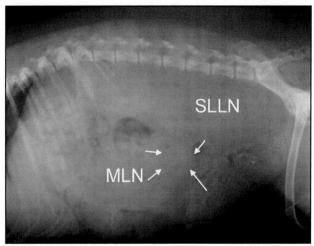

Figure 7-6
Lateral view of an older male Pomeranian with a testicular mass in a retained testicle (arrows). The dog also had enlarged mesenteric (MLN) and sublumbar lymph nodes (SLLN).

Benign Prostatic Hyperplasia

✓ Caused by an increase in intercellular spaces and ducts

✓ Cysts may be present and may or may not communicate with the urethra

Roentgen Signs

✓ Caudo-ventral abdominal mass at the neck of the urinary bladder

✓ The mass will be symmetric with smooth margins unless a large cyst is present

Roentgen Signs on Urethrography

✓ Urethra will travel through center of prostate

✓ Prostatic ducts may fill normally

✓ Prostatic cysts that communicate with the urethra are smooth and oval

✓ Some prostatic cysts that do not communicate can become large and cause asymmetry

Prostatitis

Roentgen Signs

✓ Appearance is similar to that of benign prostatic hyperplasia (prostate is diffusely enlarged).

Prostatic Abscess

Roentgen Signs

✓ Can cause symmetric or asymmetric enlargement of the prostate

Prostatic Neoplasia

Roentgen Signs

✓ Caudo-ventral abdominal mass is located at the neck of the urinary bladder

♥ Mass may be asymmetric with irregular margins

✓ Check for sublumbar lymphadenopathy, because the medial iliac lymph nodes drain the pelvic region.

💣※ Remember to perform thoracic radiography to check for pulmonary metastasis.

♥ Mineralization may be seen associated with the cranial pubis, the ventral aspect of the caudal lumbar vertebrae, or the adjacent abdominal wall.

✓ The adjacent abdominal wall may be thickened.

Roentgen Signs on Urethrography

✓ Contrast may flow into large irregular cavities

✓ Cavities may be smooth-walled but they may contain masses in the lumen

Prostatic and Paraprostatic Cysts

✓ Prostatic cysts can become so large that they are no longer within the prostatic parenchyma.

✓ A true paraprostatic cyst is uterus masculinus caused by enlargement of the Muellerian ducts.

Roentgen Signs

♥ A large prostatic cyst that has become paraprostatic may resemble a urinary bladder (Figure 7-7).

✓ *Uterus masculinus* can resemble uterine enlargement (bilateral tubular opacities)

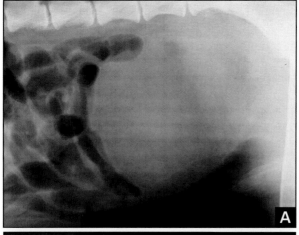

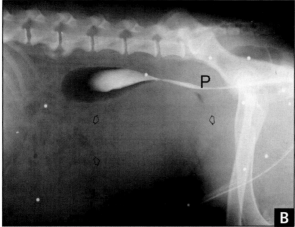

Figure 7-7
Paraprostatic cyst in a dog. **A.** Lateral view. **B.** Lateral cystogram shows the relationship of the bladder to the prostate (P) and paraprostatic cyst (arrows).

Section 8

Anomalies

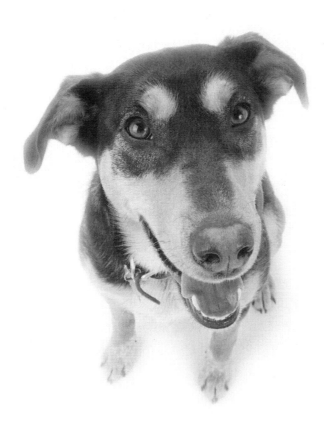

This section considers some of the more common anomalies seen in the abdomen. This type of pathology includes organs that are poorly developed, missing, or that are malpositioned.

Microhepatica

✓ Most common causes are cirrhosis and portosystemic shunt

✓ Animal may have abnormal neurologic signs, elevated bile acids, and elevated liver enzymes.

✓ Animal with cirrhosis may have a history of chronic liver disease.

✓ Animals with a portosystemic shunt are usually young and underdeveloped.

✓ Ultrasonography (especially with color flow Doppler imaging and Doppler spectral imaging) or nuclear scintigraphy should be used for further evaluation.

Roentgen Signs

✓ The gastric axis is pushed cranially.

♥ The liver mass between diaphragm and stomach is decreased (Figure 8-1). ⊙

✓ Renal and cystic calculi are common with portosystemic shunts

Renal Agenesis

✓ Apart from the reproductive organs (necessary for the survival of the species), most organs are necessary for life.

✓ Because of the built-in redundancy of the kidneys, one can be absent without abnormal clinical signs.

Roentgen Signs

✓ One kidney is not visible in either view (Figure 8-2).

✓ Remember that only the caudal pole of the right kidney is normally seen in dogs.

✓ One or both kidneys may not be apparent in normal animals because of superimposed bowel loops.

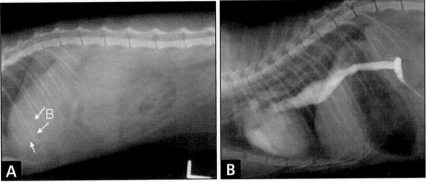

Figure 8-1
A. Lateral radiograph of a dog with a portosystemic shunt shows a small liver. Arrows indicate margins of the liver. B:gastric body. **B.** Contrast placed in a jejunal vein confirms a shunt between the portal vein and caudal vena cava.

Figure 8-2
Ventrodorsal view of a dog shows that there is no left kidney between the gastric fundus (F) and the spleen (Sp).

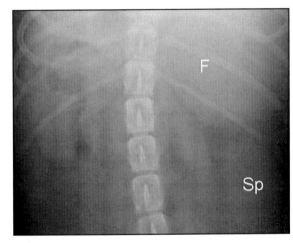

Malpositioned Kidneys

✓ One or both kidneys can be located abnormally within the abdomen.

✓ In "horseshoe" kidneys, the kidneys fail to separate into two kidneys during development.

Roentgen Signs

✓ Survey radiographs show a variably located fluid opacity.

✓ One or both renal shadows are not seen in normal position.

In a "horseshoe" kidney, one abnormally-shaped kidney is seen in an abnormal location (Figure 8-3) ⊙

✓ An excretory urogram can be performed to identify the location of the kidney(s).

Kartagener's Syndrome

✓ Here we break the rule of sticking to common diseases. All rules are made to be broken.

Kartagener's Syndrome is too interesting to ignore!

✓ In this syndrome, there are sinus and bronchial abnormalities, but the most striking abnormality is that thoracic and abdominal organs are on the wrong side of the body (situs inversus).

Roentgen Signs

✓ It is not unusual to argue as to whether the film was correctly labeled or not.

✓ In some cases, the films were re-labeled and the truth discovered during ultrasonography.

♥ Films are the mirror image of what is expected (Figure 8-4).

Figure 8-3

Radiographs of a cat with a "horseshoe" kidney. **A.** Lateral survey radiograph shows an opacity in the caudoventral abdomen superimposed over the urinary bladder. Notice that neither kidney is visible in normal position. **B.** Close-up lateral view. **C.** A cystogram identifies the urinary bladder. A second opacity (arrows) remains visible. **D.** An excretory urogram identifies the opacity as a "horseshoe" kidney. UB:urinary bladder. Radiographs are courtesy of Needham Animal Hospital, Wilmington, North Carolina.

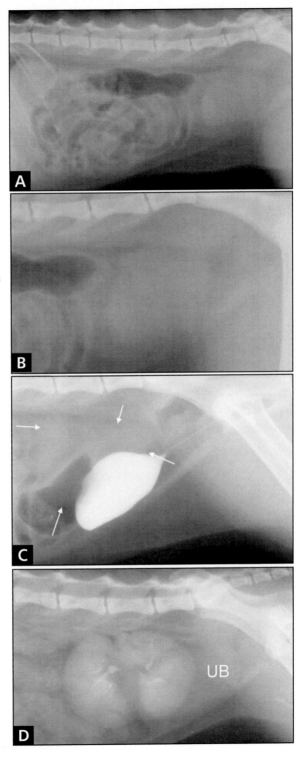

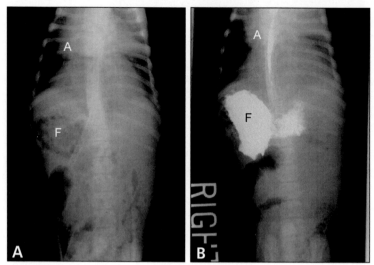

Figure 8-4
Ventrodorsal views of a dog with Kartagener's syndrome. A:cardiac apex. F:gastric fundus. **A.** Survey radiograph suggests situs inversus. Ingesta is in the gastric fundus. **B.** Barium was placed in the stomach and the film was carefully labeled to confirm the condition. The cardiac apex and gastric fundus are located on the right side.